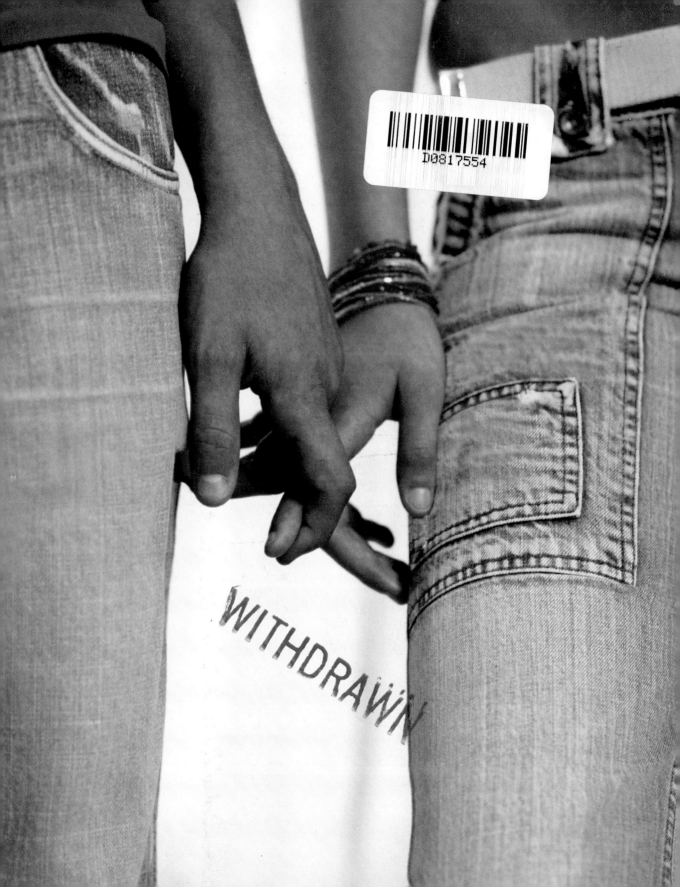

WITHDRAWN

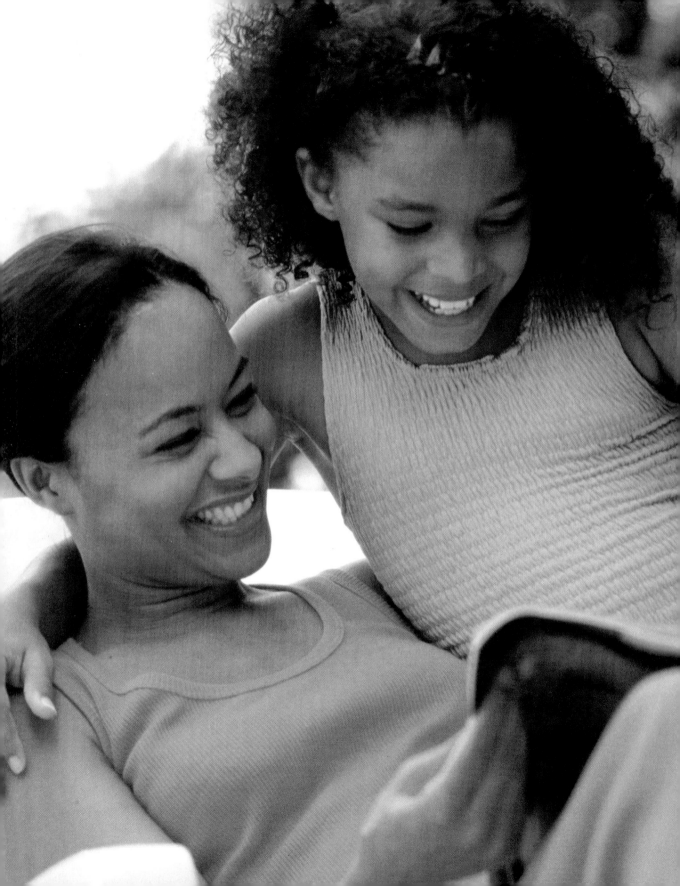

Talking to YOUR kids about SEX

Turning "the talk" into A CONVERSATION FOR LIFE

DR. LAURA BERMAN

Contents

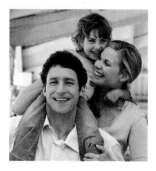
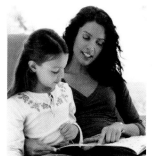
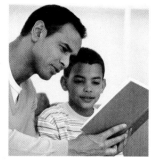
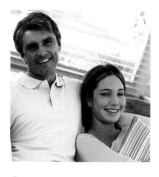

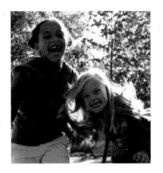
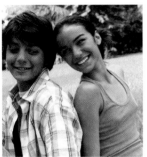
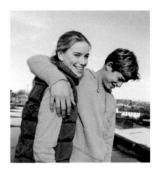
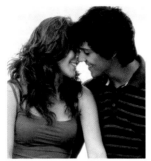

Teaching sexual truth

"Mommy, where do babies come from?"

For centuries, this question has struck fear in the hearts of parents everywhere. How can you begin to explain the complexities, the intricacies, and the very adult world of sex to a child whose primary interests are cartoons and stuffed animals? Is it even appropriate to begin to explain sometimes scary sexual truths to someone who doesn't know that Santa Claus is make-believe?

In the wake of such questions, it is no surprise that many parents opt to keep sexual knowledge hidden under lock and key. We assume that we are doing so in our children's best interests—to protect them from life's adult realities, and perhaps from the very reality of growing up. Or, maybe, just maybe, we want to keep them kids for as long as possible. We don't want to give up cuddling and butterfly kisses for the birds-and-the-bees talk. And so, our children grow up much the way we did: hearing about sex in the schoolyard; learning half-truths and urban legends; and, eventually, discovering sex through their own experiences (for better or worse).

Empowering Children

Although this lack of sex education has created a myriad of problems for past generations, it is only recently that we have truly seen the tragic results of ignorance: One in four teenage girls in the United States has an STD. The national teen pregnancy rate has increased for the first time in decades. Indeed, 1 in 5 American teens has sex by age 15, and 1 in 3 girls are pregnant by age 20. Chlamydia and syphilis have also increased across the board. And, although the emotional toll of early sexual activity isn't as easy to calculate, 60 percent of sexually active teens admit to regretting their first time, which can lead to low self-esteem, shame, and depression.

It is clear that a lack of sex education does not promote abstinence or safer sex practices. We know this because national teen pregnancy rates declined after the implementation of sexual education classes in all public schools. However, these numbers flat-lined, and then slowly increased once the focus returned to abstinence-only education. Instead of teaching kids how to protect their bodies and how to navigate birth control concerns, we started teaching them "just say no" and "sex is bad." Yet fear tactics only work for so long, especially with naturally curious, hormonally driven teens who live in a world that features sexual imagery everywhere. And when you teach children, even subconsciously, that sex is bad and that they should be ashamed or frightened of their natural sexual urges, it causes them to place a low worth on their sexuality and their bodies—which can lead to a lifetime of sexual difficulties and poor sexual choices. Of course, that doesn't mean that we shouldn't try to do all we can to protect our children from the sometimes harsh consequences of sexual activity. However, we can't protect them without empowering them with the information and confidence they need to keep themselves safe.

Empowering Parents

Unfortunately, helping children learn about sex is often unguided. Many parents end up repeating the lessons they learned when they were children, although those lessons were incomplete and uncomfortable. This book is written with these parents—with every parent—in mind. Not only will it get you thinking about larger issues surrounding sexuality (such as healthy body image and positive self-esteem), but it will also help you understand what your child needs to learn from you about sex at each stage of childhood.

This book is not meant to replace your own religious or moral beliefs about sex, or to change your views on parenting and supervision for your child. At every stage, it is meant to guide you as you communicate your personal beliefs and your family's sexual values. This begins with talking about the body, including accurate anatomy and knowledge about gender, and moves through all the major topics related to sex and sexual health: the mind and how you perceive sexuality; the media and how you absorb sexual information; friends and how they influence you; early romantic relationships; and, finally, the realities of sexual relationships and safer sex.

Using this book

Throughout this book, the references to 'he' and 'she' are meant to be used interchangeably. Unless information is specific to girls (how to use a tampon) or specific to boys (nocturnal emissions), every part of this book can be shared with both genders. A key point about a comprehensive sex education is that girls and boys should learn the same things. This means that your son should know how a girl's body works, and your daughter should understand how a boy's body works. This can help remove the mystery from sex, and makes it easier to transition into more complex sexual lessons as your child grows. And despite traditional stereotypes, information on a healthy body image and sexual protection and pregnancy is as relevant to boys as to girls, and information on self-stimulation and open communication is as relevant to girls as to boys.

As you read, you will find interactive pages labeled "Learning Together," which can be looked at with your child. These include step-by-step lesson plans on important topics; answers to "big" questions your child might have; and, in some cases, anatomical or instructive diagrams. In addition, "Teachable Moment" boxes throughout the book help identify natural moments to bring up sexual issues, Q&A panels provide answers to common questions kids ask, and "What to Say" boxes walk you through how to handle difficult conversations. Additionally, sample dialogue is highlighted in bold throughout the book to maximize the potential for healthy conversation.

Having these conversations can change your child's sexual future, and can also impact social outlook and self-esteem. Not only will talking openly about sex help keep your child as safe as possible, it will also help to deepen your bond and improve your communication, making your relationship a source of support and unconditional love for your child.

Enjoy!

Laura Berman

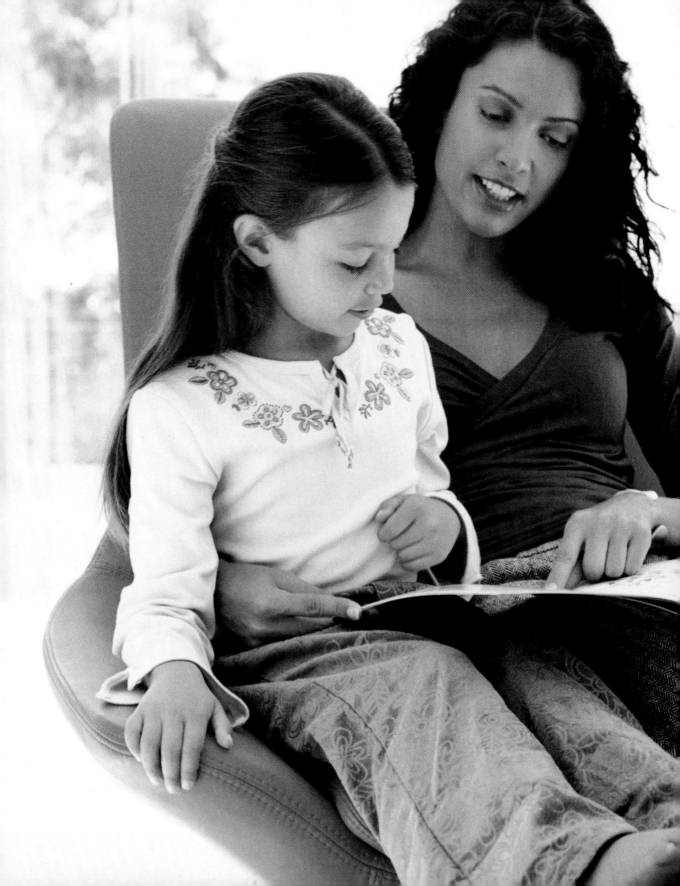

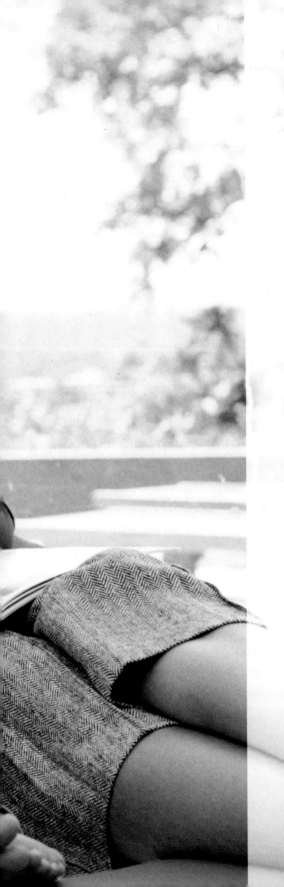

1

TALKING ABOUT THE BODY

ASSESSING YOUR VALUES: THE BODY

So many factors influence the way we feel about our bodies. These can be conscious or unconscious—either way they will be passed down to your child as you talk about anatomy and sexual health. The first step in deciding your values is to think about your own influences and insecurities. Next, think about when you want your child to learn certain facts. Answer these questions privately, then reflect with your partner on how to blend your views to give your child a healthy understanding of the body.

EXPLORING THE BODY

Identifying your thoughts and feelings about your body will illuminate any insecurities so that you can make a conscious effort not to pass these on to your child.

How do you view your own body? Is it a source of pride, discomfort, or worry?

What do you love about your body?

What would you change about your body?

How do you care for your body?

When do you think is the appropriate time to learn about the genitals?

What terms did you use growing up to describe your genitals?

Have you ever worried about the appearance of your genitals? Do you think it is important to feel good about your genitals?

What early lessons did you learn about the body (spoken or unspoken)? Were you taught to be open about the body or to cover it up? How has this influenced the way you think about the body as an adult?

When did you first learn about conception and birth, and how did this knowledge impact you?

EXPLORING GOOD AND BAD TOUCH

Think about how you value touch, and about what types of touch you find inappropriate. Reflect equally on good types of touch that show affection or help you to understand and appreciate your body better.

What types of touch do you consider bad?

Do you think talking about inappropriate touching should be part of your child's sexual education? If so, how early do you think you should have this talk?

How important do you think affectionate touch is, and what role does it play in defining your self-esteem and your relationships?

How physically affectionate are you and your partner in public and in front of your child?

What things make you uncomfortable as your child starts to explore the body?

Do you think masturbation is appropriate as a form of sexual release?

Do you think masturbation should be discussed as part of a child's education?

How would you respond if you saw your young child touching the genitals in public? Would you be embarrassed, worried, or calm?

EXPLORING GENDER

Lessons about gender are often passed along subconsciously. Think about how you view the body of the opposite sex, and why this is so.

When did you learn about the body of the opposite sex?

What do you think are the primary differences between boys and girls?

How would you react if you found your child "playing doctor" or exploring the body with a friend of the opposite gender?

Would you feel uncomfortable if your child began to enjoy activities that were typically reserved for the opposite gender, such as if your son wanted to play dress up regularly or paint his nails?

Do you remember your earliest friendship with the opposite sex? How did it impact you?

EXPLORING LIFESTYLE

Consider what lifestyle choices—both present and future—will encourage a healthy body image from an early age, and will help fulfill your hopes for your child's self-esteem and sex life, both during adolescence and adulthood.

What physical components are essential for a healthy lifestyle? What value do you place on sleep, exercise, nutrition, and affection?

What do you think the relationship is between a healthy body image and healthy, responsible sexual behavior? Have you noticed this connection in your own life?

What lifestyle habits did you grow up believing to be important? How have they continued to impact you as an adult?

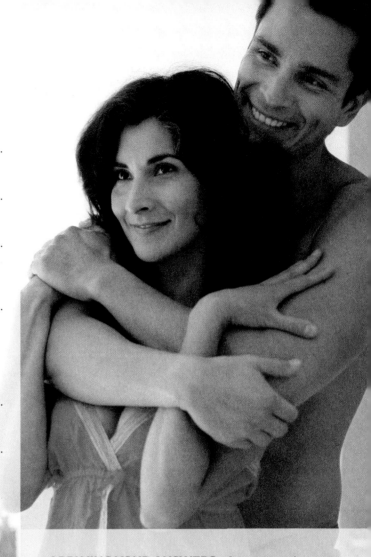

APPLYING YOUR ANSWERS After answering these questions, you may feel comfortable addressing these issues with your child. Or, you might realize that there are topics that will be difficult to discuss. Many of us have mental scripts from childhood that still play in our head, which make us anxious about sex or our bodies. Answering these questions is the first step in discovering these scripts, and replacing old harmful messages with new empowering ones. Simply becoming aware of any mental roadblocks will put you in a more peaceful place as you begin your child's sexual education.

Your child's physical development

Children develop physically and gain sexual knowledge from the day they are born, though of course they are not truly sexual in the adult sense of the word. Exploring the body, asking about gender, and reveling in nakedness are all normal and natural for young children. By understanding the stages of awareness and behavior you will be able to plan for and anticipate your child's needs.

Your child's sexual awareness

Sexual awareness and behavior develop slowly at first, perhaps so slowly that you don't even notice it. Over time, you will see more changes, as your child grows fully into his identity and sexuality. Being prepared for this process can help you nurture your child during each stage.

0–2 years old. Your child touches her genitals and might even stimulate herself. This is even true for babies who are only three to five months old. Why do they do this? Quite simply, because it feels good and is soothing. This type of touch is not unnatural.

2–5 years old. By age 2, your child will have noticed that men and women are different, even if he doesn't fully grasp what these differences are. By age 3, your child will have developed a clear gender identity. Many children of this age like to be naked, which is completely natural. Your child will probably still enjoy touching his genitals, although he may now restrict this behavior to the home. Introductory questions about the body and sex become common.

6–9 years old. During this stage, a child's understanding of sex develops to include knowledge about the basic mechanics of sex. Kissing and other adult behavior in movies or in real life causes embarrassment, but also triggers curiosity. Your child will also begin to wonder about the opposite gender's body, and may play the "I'll show you mine, if you'll show me yours" game. This is healthy, provided your child is not touching or being touched by other children or acting sexually inappropriately, which can be a sign of abuse.

10–12 years old. Your child may become highly embarrassed or anxious about his body. Pre-adolescents are entering a stage when they can understand more detailed mechanics and emotional implications of sex, and for most, it makes them curious and sometimes scared. He will also become very interested in the opposite sex and may have his first romantic relationship. Talking to your child openly about changes, feelings, and insecurities can help him feel more comfortable during this time.

12–19 years old. Your child is growing into an adult and enters her own sexual awakening. During this time, children often become fascinated with things of a sexual nature, and discovering sexual stimulation becomes compelling. Self-stimulation is common and healthy during this time. Interest in romantic relationships increases, and these relationships may become sexual. Your child will need to learn about STDs, contraception, and the emotional responsibility that goes hand in hand with these physical concerns.

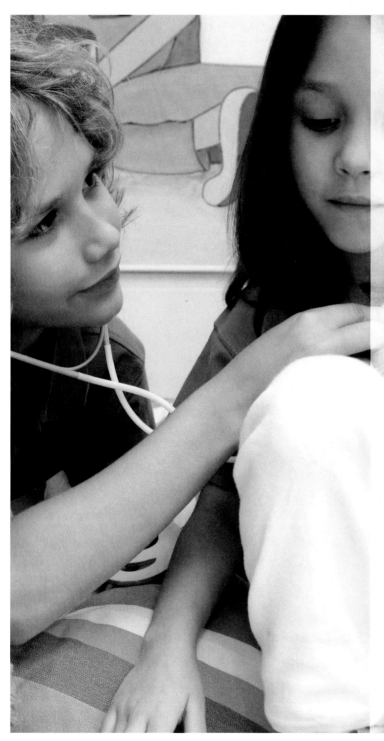

WHAT TO SAY . . .
IF YOUR CHILD IS UNCOMFORTABLE WITH HIS CHANGING BODY

....

It is not uncommon for your child to experience some discomfort or insecurity as his body changes. This could happen during puberty, or earlier on as he grows. If you feel he is an anxious or insecure about his body, support him by having an open conversation about these changes.

CONVERSATION STARTER: "You might be feeling a little self-conscious with the changes with your body lately. I started feeling this way when I was around 8 years old."

Allow your child some time to respond, then go into more detail.

FOLLOW-UP: "I felt like I was living in someone else's body. But, after a few months passed, I started to get more accustomed to the changes that were happening to me, inside and out."

If your child continues to feel anxious, have a follow-up conversation.

CONVERSATION STARTER "I know it might seem like you are the only one who is feeling this way, but I promise you everyone feels insecure about their body sometimes. Many of your classmates might feel this way, too."

Once you have normalized these feelings, make sure your child knows that you are always open to talk.

FOLLOW-UP: "I hope you know that you can come talk to me any time. I know what it is like to have doubts and insecurities and I am here to answer all of your questions."

Teaching about the body

It is a good idea to teach your child about the body from a young age. Using accurate language and being relaxed about the body's functions will help encourage a healthy body image. Provide age-appropriate information and stay attuned to your child's natural curiosity and she will cultivate a healthy respect for her body.

Using accurate language

It is important to use the proper terms for all of your child's body parts from infancy. This includes using accurate terms for the genitals. The correct term for the female genitals is "vulva." (Medically speaking, "vagina" is only used in reference to the actual vaginal canal, not the whole of the female genital anatomy.) The correct terms for the male genitalia are "penis" and "testes."

As you teach your child these terms, also take into account the common words that children his age use. For example, as you explain the vulva, mention that some people call this the vagina, and that although that word refers more specifically to the vaginal cavity, when other children say this they will generally mean the female genitals. Explain that this is a common misunderstanding and that while he can use either phrase and does not need to correct his friends, "vulva" is the correct term.

If you don't generally use the proper terms in reference to your own body, it will likely take some time to feel comfortable using them with your child. However, it is important that you take this step. Using cute nicknames for our genitals or those of our children sends the message that the genitals are embarrassing or silly or uncomfortable. Just like your child has an elbow, a shoulder, and a nose, he or she also has a penis or a vulva. If you use these terms from day one, your child will be less likely to feel embarrassment or awkwardness when talking about the genitals.

Using accurate language from the start also means that your child will feel confident enough later in life to openly discuss health concerns

>>> YOUR CHILD IS READY TO TALK ABOUT THE GENITALS WHEN...

The two-year mark is generally a good time to begin talking about the genitals, though it may be earlier or later, depending on your child's development. This first conversation will likely be one of many that you will have, as it often takes children time to fully grasp and retain the information. Signs that your child is ready to begin talking about the genitals include:

• Exploring the genitals on a semi-regular basis
• Asking questions about the body
• Expressing curiosity about the bodies of others

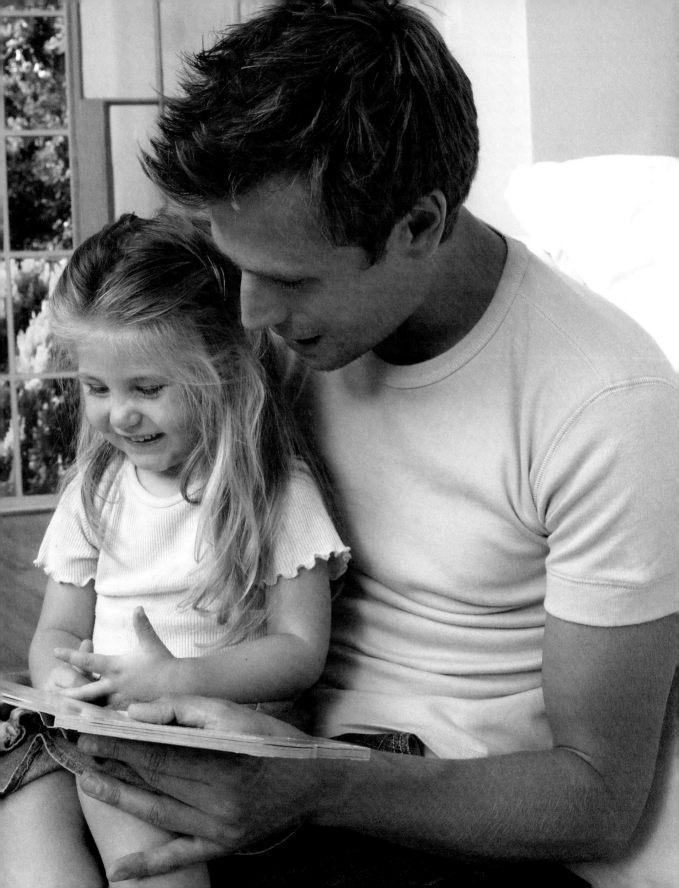

with a doctor. In addition, using correct terminology can help better protect your child from inappropriate sexual contact, as he will understand his own genitals and will be less likely to feel any shame or confusion when talking to you about his body.

Discussing bodily functions

Even for adults, bodily functions often cause cringes or giggles—and understandably so. The body can act in ways that are strange, embarrassing, and unpredictable. However, it is important that you move beyond these reflex reactions and take the time to demystify and normalize the body's functions for your child.

If you don't do this, your child might end up feeling embarrassed or ashamed of her body, or unable to open up to you about any concerns, particularly concerns about genital pain. For example, many little girls are prone to urinary tract infections, which are sometimes triggered by bubble baths. If your daughter doesn't feel comfortable coming to you and explaining that it hurts when she uses the bathroom, her health could be at risk. This is why it is important that your child understands and feels comfortable with all of her bodily functions—so that when something does go wrong, she can feel safe expressing this to you.

You can help your child achieve this feeling of comfort and safety by not overreacting to bodily functions. Many parents tend to feel uncomfortable or even revolted while changing diapers or helping their child in the bathroom, and they let these feelings show. Negative comments or expressions send a clear message to your child—her bodily functions are gross!

Make an effort to avoid negative messages by saying "What a healthy bowel movement!" when changing your child or helping to wipe them. This will teach your child that bodily functions are natural and healthy—a lesson that will also help her feel confident about the rest of her body.

Keeping information age-appropriate

As your child grows, he will naturally have questions about the body that move beyond simply naming physical parts. He might begin to ask "Why do I have bumps on my tongue?", or questions more difficult to answer, such as "Why does my penis sometimes become hard?"

If you pause and think of how to answer these questions in an age-appropriate way, they will lose much of their intimidation factor. Giving age-appropriate information simply means talking about the body in a way that fits the age and maturity level of your child. The best way to determine what information your child is ready to know is to think about the type of questions he is asking. If the question is purely physical like the ones above, you can give a purely physical answer, such as: "Your penis becomes hard when there is a change in blood flow. This is natural, and can happen for no particular reason." If he is still curious, or asks questions that move beyond anatomical facts, you can continue to provide small pieces of information that answer the specific question and nothing more.

"Giving age-appropriate information simply means talking about the body in a way that fits the age and maturity level of your child."

TEACHABLE MOMENTS
TALKING ABOUT THE GENITALS

Look for these moments from an early age, starting when your child is 0–2 years old. Even before your child can talk, you can begin teaching the proper names of the genitals. Continue these conversations as your child grows and begins to ask questions. Always choose an intimate, relaxed setting where both of you feel comfortable.

• **AT THE CHANGING TABLE:** Changing your baby's diaper is a good moment for your first conversation about private parts. When your baby girl starts to play with her genitals on the changing table, you can mention, "That's your vulva." This will ensure that your child is already familiar with the correct anatomical language as she grows up.

• **IN THE TUB:** Bath time is a good moment for a follow-up conversation. Your child will be relaxed, and will already be looking at his own body, perhaps even vocalizing thoughts and questions about what he sees. Begin by talking about larger limbs and body parts, and asking your child the correct name for each. From there, it is easy and natural to transition into talking about the genitals. Point to this part of the body, and ask your child "Do you know what we call that? That's your penis. Boys have penises and girls have vulvas. That's part of what makes boys and girls different."

• **DURING PLAYTIME:** As your child grows older, she might begin to touch her private parts frequently, sometimes in public settings, such as at school or when playing with other children. This is a natural method of self-soothing, but to save yourself and your child embarrassment, it is best to have a conversation about how genitals are private parts. Pull her aside in the moment or later in the day and gently say something such as, "It feels good to touch your private parts, doesn't it? That is normal, but remember that because they are private, it is best to touch them in private, too."

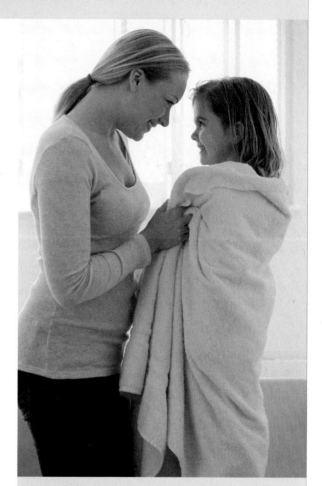

CONVERSATION STARTER 1: "Let's name the parts of your body. This is your nose. This is your elbow. This is your ankle. This is your knee. This is your vulva. Do you know what to call all of these parts?"

CONVERSATION STARTER 2: "Your genitals are a special and unique part of your body. Do you know where these are? Do you have any questions about them?"

Learning together

LEARNING ABOUT PARTS OF THE BODY

Teaching your child about his body encourages him to respect and take care of it. A good time to start doing this is when your child is between the ages of 4 and 6. Boys and girls should learn the proper names and functions for the parts of the body of both genders so that they don't develop embarrassment about either the male or female body. If you like, you can have your child draw these images afterward to make sure he is comfortable with the terms and parts and can remember them without prompting.

AFTER THIS LESSON, YOUR CHILD WILL BE MORE LIKELY TO...

- Feel comfortable, secure, and relaxed about his body
- Find it easy to talk to you about pain in the genital area
- Remember that his genitals are private and should only be touched by himself or a caretaker in private
- Be protected against sexual predators who target children that don't feel in control of their bodies
- Take responsibility for his own body, including health and safety
- Develop a healthy body image as he moves into adolescence.

---

1 WHAT ARE THE PARTS OF THE BODY?
Ask your child to touch and name all the parts of the body that he knows about. These should be non-private parts to start. If your child has trouble beginning, you can help by pointing to a specific part of the body and asking the name. Talking about the non-sexual parts of the body first will help you both feel more comfortable and relaxed as you begin.

2 ARE THERE ANY PARTS WE HAVEN'T NAMED?
Once you have named all of these parts, ask your child if there are any parts that weren't named. Give your child a chance to answer, then say, "The other parts of the body are your private parts. These are the parts that you don't see or touch in public. Boys and girls have different private parts." Your child may start to giggle at this point, which is normal and expected. Let him know that adults often giggle about these private parts, too, but that they are unique and special parts of the body that should be talked about and understood.

3 WHAT ARE YOUR PRIVATE PARTS?
Show your child the diagram for his own gender, and point to the genitals. Describe each part using the proper name, and say how it works. Point to the penis and the testes, and explain that these are where sperm is created. Tell your child that this is one of the ways that the male body is unique and different from the female body. Reiterate that these parts are special and private and should be kept private. Ask your child if he has any questions about his body, or how any of the male parts work.

4 WHAT ARE THE OTHER SEX'S PRIVATE PARTS?
Show your child the diagram for the female body. Go into the same detail about each part and say that these parts are equally private and special. Explain how the female body has breasts and curves, which make it is the perfect environment for a baby to grow. Talk about the vulva, and let your child know that this special part of the female genitals also houses the vaginal opening, which is where a baby comes out. Once you finish, go back over the diagrams with your child and ask him to tell you about each part of the genitals, both male and female. If your child seems shy, you can prompt him as you did in the begining by pointing to parts of the body and asking that he tell you about that part.

THE FEMALE BODY

THE MALE BODY

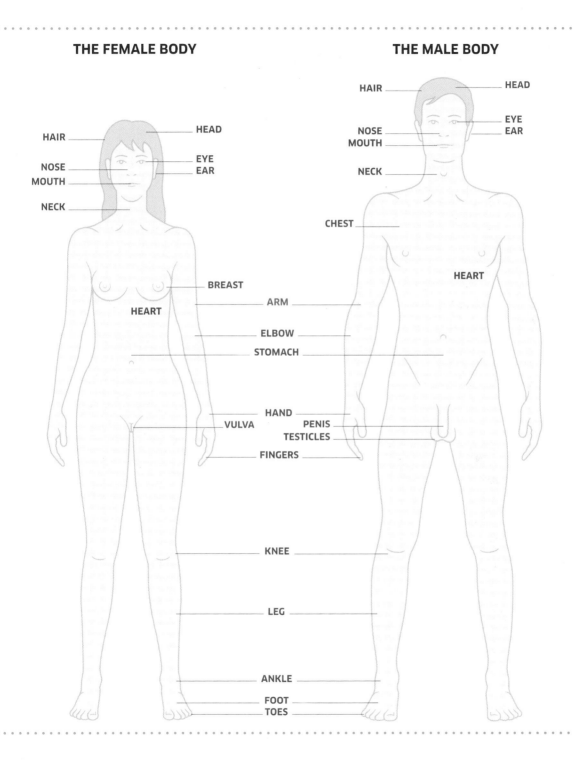

HAIR

HEAD

NOSE
MOUTH

EYE
EAR

NECK

CHEST

HEART

HAIR

HEAD

NOSE

EYE
EAR

MOUTH

NECK

HEART

BREAST

ARM

ELBOW

STOMACH

HAND

VULVA

PENIS
TESTICLES

FINGERS

KNEE

LEG

ANKLE

FOOT
TOES

Learning together

Explaining gender differences

Gender is one of the first "sexual" topics your child will be deeply curious about. Society often focuses on strict gender differences, but if you teach more flexible lessons about gender your child will be more likely to feel at ease with her unique personality and to grow into a confident and accepting adult.

Early gender behavior

Around the ages of 3-4, your child will start to notice gender behavior and will begin to play out gender roles. Strong likes and dislikes for toys and activities will begin to emerge, often driven by a need to play out the correct gender role, and hence gain approval. Of course, your child does not think these thoughts consciously, but he does notice that, for instance, Daddy likes to play football and that Mommy likes to cook, and he will start to imitate "correct" behavior in order to fit into the family's mold.

Make it a point to have open gender roles. Perhaps Daddy helps cook meals, and Mommy shows an interest in sports, too. This open environment will help your child feel less stressed and anxious over his own gender behavior, and will encourage your child's true personality traits and interests to emerge.

Understanding gender scripts

Many gender scripts and stereotypes begin from a very early age. In fact, as you read some of the common gender scripts, you might think to yourself, "But my girlfriends and I really do like to shop and talk on the phone!" or "It is true that I hate to talk about my feelings." However, consider that one of the reasons you identify with certain gender-specific behaviors is because you learned from a very young age that these were the types of behaviors you were meant to enjoy. In other words, as a young girl, you might have helped out your mother in the kitchen or accompanied her on shopping errands. Now, decades later, you might still love to cook, bake and shop—because as a young child, those activities made you feel close to your mother. You were playing out your "appropriate" role, from which you gained confidence and self-esteem.

However, the truth is that anatomy alone does not dictate these interests. Girls can love sports and cars, just like boys can love cooking and playing house. Even though many parents now know and accept the fact that gender-specific behavior is not genetic or natural, we still tend to raise children based around these simple gender definitions. If you can discard these in favor of a more fluid understanding of gender, your child will grow up to be a more open and confident individual, and will feel free to fully explore her unique personality and identity, rather than subscribing to a strict set of rules.

Encouraging gender exploration

One reason that parents promote traditional gender roles is that it is easy. There are plenty of dolls and pink baby clothes to be found at the mall for a baby girl, but not many sports-themed or interactive gifts. The opposite is true for a baby boy. We also encourage these roles because we want our children to be accepted, and to have active social lives and plenty of friends. Realistically, we don't live in a society that accepts a boy who loves baking and sewing as easily as a boy who likes video games and skateboarding. Because of this, we guide our children toward behaviors that will make them feel accepted, and toward activities that are typical for their gender.

This is not the healthiest approach, however. The confidence that comes from being part of an open and accepting household can be more lasting and substantial than the confidence that comes from easy peer acceptance. Empowering children to be confident enough to forge their own identity and go after their dreams, regardless of outdated gender scripts, is a lifelong gift. Additionally, it is becoming more common for children to grow up in homes that encourage less strict gender definitions, which means that your child is more likely to have peers that are part of similarly open families. Non-traditional gender behavior does not threaten social happiness in the way it once did.

So, the next time your son wants to play with his sister's dolls, or your daughter wants to play football, don't overreact. The less you react, the more comfortable and safe your child will feel acting in a way which is natural to them. Your child's behavior may or may not change over time, but it is important to realize that you can't control how your child chooses to express his gender, and that the most loving and helpful thing to do is to support him as he seeks out his own interests.

Dealing with gender confusion

While most gender experimentation is completely harmless, there are certain signs that indicate your child might be dealing with gender confusion. If your child insists that she is of the   opposite gender, and possibly even asks to be treated as such, this is a sign that serious confusion may exist. Under these circumstances,

SEXPLANATION
WHAT IS GENDER SCRIPTING?

"Gender scripting" is the term used to define human behavior that is dictated by gender roles. In other words, when children follow a gender script, they determine their actions and words based on what society has told them boys and girls are supposed to do. Typical gender scripts include:

- Girls aren't good at math and science.
- Boys are good at sports.
- Girls are good listeners.
- Boys don't cry.
- Girls are emotional.
- Boys don't like talking about their feelings.
- Girls like to shop and talk on the phone.
- Boys like to watch television.
- Girls like to play dress-up and wear makeup.
- Boys like to play video games.
- Girls should be quiet and well-mannered.
- Boys are hyperactive and like to roughhouse.

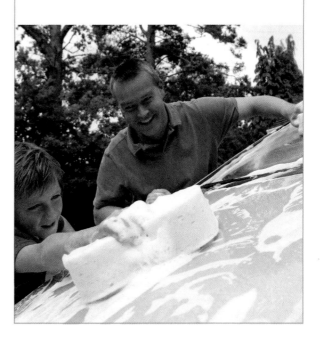

your child will often withdraw socially, experience anxiety, and have a hard time making friends. If you think there is an issue, seek the help of a trained child therapist—if possible, one who specializes in gender issues.

Not every case of gender rejection points to a deeper issue. Sometimes children reject their own gender as a way of dealing with anxiety around sexual development. If your preadolescent daughter has been teased at school about her growing breasts, or your son is feeling like he can't keep up with the sports his peers are playing at recess, it is not uncommon to begin to temporarily identify with the opposite gender. Only further exploration and therapy can identify the true cause of the issue. In the meantime, remaining judgment-free is the best tool you have to help your child comfortably navigate gender identity or sexual identity considerations.

Talking about the body of the opposite sex

The opposite sex is often a mystery to us, even during childhood. Around the same time that children begin noticing gender roles, they will often begin asking questions such as "Mommy, why do boys have a penis?" or "Why do girls have breasts and boys don't?" These questions can be uncomfortable and alarming the first time they come up, but remember that they don't reflect any true sexual interest. Children want to know about the anatomy of the opposite sex not only to satisfy their curiosity about their peers, but also to satisfy their growing curiosity about their own bodies.

By demystifying the anatomy of the opposite sex from an early age, you can keep your child informed and satisfy his natural curiosity, removing some of the need for the "I will show you mine if you show me yours" type of exploration. It can also continue to help establish an open environment in your home.

Define and explain both male and female anatomy as accurately as possible, using the charts and definitions from pages 24–25. It is a good idea to show your child the diagrams for both genders, and thus normalize the importance of understanding sexual anatomy for both genders. Remember that the genitals of the opposite sex will not have sexual resonance for your three-year-old in the way they would for an adult. By showing your child these charts, you are simply satisfying his curiosity about anatomy, and affirming his realization that boys and girls are physically different and special.

Gender roles in early friendships

Your child's early social interactions will not only teach her important lessons about sharing, communicating, and social behavior, it will also teach her invaluable lessons about gender behavior. Most children enjoy playing with friends of the opposite sex, sometimes well into adolescence, and sometimes just until they get "cooties" around age 8 or 9, when the earliest feelings of attraction start to set in. These friendships can be fundamental to the way your child relates to the opposite sex later in life. Children who establish opposite-sex

"Children want to know about the anatomy of the opposite sex to satisfy curiosity about their peers, as well as curiosity about their own bodies."

friendships early on are more likely to interact easily with both genders as adults, and to be more accepting of a range of gender behaviors.

In addition, your child will learn an immense amount from friends of the same gender about how she should and should not act. In fact, some of the most influential lessons about gender roles can come from early childhood friendships. For example, if your child's friends are open to exploration of gender behavior, whether or not this behavior is typically labeled as "girls only" or "boys only," your child will generally have a more fluid and authentic understanding of gender. Alternately, if your daughter has a friend who comes from a home of very strict gender behavior, she might begin to dislike all things masculine, just as her friend has been taught to do. Pay attention to your child's behavior and conversation around her friends. If your child has a friend that reinforces gender stereotypes or teases your child for having a wide range of interests, find a quiet time to sit down with your child and have a heart-to-heart talk that will reinforce your family values about gender.

You might say: "I heard [name of friend] tell you that girls like dolls, and not sports. You know that isn't true all the time, don't you? Girls can like sports and dolls, and boys can like both, too. Everybody has different things that they think are fun. That is why it is important to have new friends and try new things."

HOW TO ANSWER QUESTIONS ABOUT GENDER

Some of the earliest questions your child will ask will likely be about gender. As with all of your young child's questions about sex, aim to provide age-appropriate information by honestly answering the question without sharing too many specific details.

Q. How are boys and girls different?
A. Boys and girls have different body parts. Boys have penises and testicles and girls have vulvas and will develop breasts. But they both like a lot of the same things, and they are both equal. You can have friends who are boys and friends who are girls, and have just as much fun with either!

Q. Why do girls have breasts?
A. Women have breasts because that is how they feed their babies.

Q. Are boys stronger than girls?
A. Girls and boys have different bodies and boys are sometimes stronger, but girls can play just like boys. They can run, catch, and play sports... they can do any activity that they find interesting and fun.

Q. Are girls smarter than boys?
A. Girls sometimes perform better in school, but girls and boys are equally smart. You can learn a lot if you try hard in school, no matter if you are a boy or a girl.

Q. Why do girls wear dresses, and boys pants?
A. Some girls like to wear dresses because they think they are pretty, but girls can, and often do, wear pants, too. In the US, boys don't usually wear dresses unless they are playing dress up, but in other countries, such as Scotland or South Africa, boys have traditionally worn skirts and dresses in normal life, too.

LEARNING ABOUT GENDER DIFFERENCES

Talking about the differences between girls and boys and their reproductive organs from an early age helps avoid potential misunderstanding and embarrassment later on. Plan to hold the first discussion when your child is between the ages of 5 and 7, then return to the lesson when your child is older. As you use these diagrams to introduce the genitals to your child, it is a good idea to tell her that the diagrams shown are abstract renderings, and that to truly understand this part of her body, she can examine her own genitals and see how they look and how they function.

AFTER THIS LESSON YOUR CHILD WILL BE MORE LIKELY TO...
- Know how boys' and girls' genitals are different and why
- Be able to identify the different parts of the genitals of both sexes
- Feel more comfortable talking to you about the reproductive organs
- Have greater awareness and ownership of his or her own body and how it works
- Be less likely to be confused or worried by misinformed friends or peers.

MALE ANATOMY

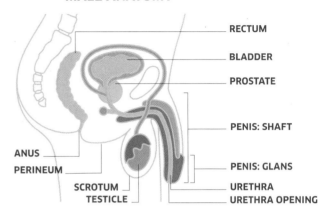

RECTUM
BLADDER
PROSTATE
PENIS: SHAFT
ANUS
PERINEUM
PENIS: GLANS
SCROTUM
TESTICLE
URETHRA
URETHRA OPENING

1   WHAT MAKES UP THE MALE GENITALS?
Ask your child to name the parts of the genitals. If she needs help, point to the testicles and explain that men have two of these, which hang just behind the penis in a bag called the scrotum. Explain that, beginning at puberty, the testicles produce tiny sperm that fertilize a woman's egg to make a baby. Point to the penis and say that it is made up of a glans and a shaft, and that it carries urine and sperm.

UNCIRCUMCISED PENIS   **CIRCUMCISED PENIS**

SHAFT
FORESKIN
GLANS

2   WHAT DOES CIRCUMCISION MEAN?
Explain that an uncircumcised penis has a foreskin, which is like a sleeve of skin over its head. The foreskin can be moved back to expose the head of the penis. Boy babies are born with a foreskin, but some are circumcised, usually as newborns, which means that the foreskin is removed. This doesn't impact the way a man urinates or passes sperm.

EXTERNAL FEMALE ANATOMY

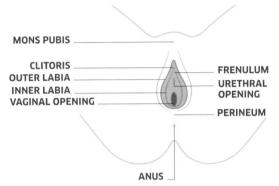

MONS PUBIS

CLITORIS
OUTER LABIA
INNER LABIA
VAGINAL OPENING

FRENULUM
URETHRAL OPENING
PERINEUM

ANUS

INTERNAL FEMALE ANATOMY

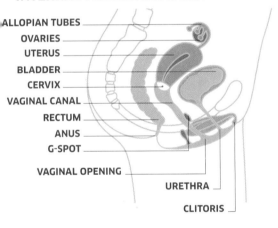

FALLOPIAN TUBES
OVARIES
UTERUS
BLADDER
CERVIX
VAGINAL CANAL
RECTUM
ANUS
G-SPOT
VAGINAL OPENING

URETHRA
CLITORIS

ANATOMY OF THE BREAST

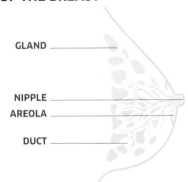

GLAND

NIPPLE
AREOLA

DUCT

3 WHICH PARTS OF THE FEMALE GENITALS CAN YOU SEE?

Help your child identify the outer labia, the inner labia, the clitoris, the vagina, and the urethral opening. Explain that the clitoris is a bump that sits at the top of the inner labia, which is filled with nerve endings. Explain also how a woman has three "holes": a urethra, where urine comes out; her vagina, where menstruation comes out and perhaps a baby; and her anus, where her bowel movements exit.

4 WHICH PARTS OF THE FEMALE GENITALS CAN'T BE SEEN?

Point to the ovaries and explain that a woman has one on each side of her uterus. They contain up to one million eggs, which she is born with. Starting at puberty, an egg travels down the fallopian tube every month. Show her where the uterus is and tell her that this is where a baby grows. Point out the cervix, which is the entrance to the uterus, and the vaginal canal, which leads up to it. When your child is older, you can explain that the g-spot, like the clitoris, is a pleasure point that feels good when stimulated.

5 WHAT ARE BREASTS FOR?

Ask your child why women have breasts and men don't. If she needs help, explain that women make milk to feed babies. Point out the glands and explain that these develop as girls grow. Each gland has a duct at the end, where milk is stored. These ducts are located in the darker area around the nipple, called the areola. When an infant sucks on the nipple, milk comes out. Breasts also contain fatty tissue, which gives them a soft shape. After you've talked about sex with an older child, you can explain that the nipples are rich in nerve endings and both men and women may find stimulation of the nipples pleasurable.

Learning together

Teaching about inappropriate touch

One of the most important aspects of sexual education is explaining the difference between good touch and bad touch. This will give your child confidence to know how his body should be treated, and will also help protect against molestation. If you talk openly about this delicate topic from the start, your child will be more likely to feel safe coming to you with concerns at any age.

Keeping the communication lines open

Talking about inappropriate touch should be an ongoing conversation that you have with your child, not a one-time conversation. This means that you don't have to feel compelled or pressured to cram this big talk into one discussion. It also means that your child will receive consistent, reliable information on a very important subject. When children aren't given the correct information from their parents about good touch and bad touch, molesters can manipulate their ignorance and feed them lies such as: "You asked for it; it's your fault" or "If you tell anyone, you will get in big trouble."

Another benefit of giving your child small pieces of information is that you can do so without scaring her or leading her to mistrust others. Starting from the time that your child is able to understand—generally around 2 or 3 years old—begin talking about how her genitals are her private parts. Emphasize that no one is allowed to touch them besides her, her parents, her doctor, and other caretakers when helping her in the bathroom. Also let her know that if she feels uncomfortable about the way a caretaker touches her, she should tell you about it right away.

Once you've established that private parts should not be touched by others, you can say in your next conversation: "If someone touches you in a way that scares you or makes you unhappy, you can come to me, no matter what. I will never be mad at you for talking to me about someone touching you or hurting you. You can always feel safe talking to me about this." Then, answer any questions or address any concerns that your child might have, and once she is satisfied, move on to a lighter topic.

A few months later, you might say "Remember when I talked to you about how these are your private parts and how no one should touch them but you? Don't forget that if anyone touches you on your private parts that you can come to me. I will always listen and I will never be angry with you." This will help reinforce the message to your child.

Although this is a difficult conversation to have, it is a good idea to reinforce it often. The more your child hears this message, the more likely it will be to sink in. In addition, your child will process and understand these messages differently at different ages. When you stress this message throughout her childhood, she will be able to understand it at a deeper level each time, and thus protect herself better.

Inappropriate touch with friends

It is a good idea to talk with your child about how these rules also apply when playing with friends. While many show-and-tell games are inevitable and reflect only typical curiosity, some children do prey upon other children sexually due to molestation in their homes or personal lives. Because of this, it is important to emphasize to your child that even friends should not touch his private parts, and that, likewise, he should not touch friends' private parts under any circumstances.

To start this conversation, you might say: "I noticed you and [friend's name] playing doctor during your play date earlier today, and I want you to know that is normal. The body is interesting to learn about. However, remember that no one should ever touch your private parts. This means that you should never touch your friend's genitals, and your friend should never touch yours."

Non-sexual inappropriate touching

These same rules apply to other kinds of unwanted touch. Perhaps your son is complaining that his playmate keeps hugging him, or your daughter is frustrated because her sister pushed her. It is important to clarify that any type of unwanted touch is unnecessary, inappropriate, and should be stopped.

For example, say to your child: "Tell your friend [sibling] that you don't want to be hugged." Stand there with him as he does so, and say to the other child, "When someone tells you they don't want to

be hugged or pushed or touched in any way, it means you have to stop. And if anyone treats you in a way you don't like, tell him or her that it needs to stop. If the other person doesn't listen, make sure to tell one of your grown-ups and we will help you."

Protecting against inappropriate touch

As your child grows, one of the best ways to protect him from possible danger is to stay aware of what's going on around you and to trust your instincts. Only seven percent of children are molested by a stranger—so while it may seem unthinkable for a family friend or a relative to harm your child, this is a sad reality for many families. Remain alert even when someone you know very well is watching your child.

Beware of someone who seems overly interested in your child, especially if this is expressed in ways that are "touchy-feely." Sexual predators often use words such as "back rub" or "massage" to make children believe that their touch is harmless, so reiterate frequently to your child that certain parts of the body should never be touched by others and that you always want to know about any type of touch that feels uncomfortable, even if it is on an "acceptable" part of the body. If your child seems to feel shy or uncomfortable around a friend, don't be afraid to speak up or remove your child from the situation.

"Talking about inappropriate touch should be an ongoing conversation that you have with your child, not a one-time conversation. This means that you don't have to feel pressured to cram this big talk into one discussion."

Date rape and acquaintance rape

If your child has been exposed to lessons about inappropriate touch from early childhood, she might be better equipped to protect herself as a teenager. Still, date and acquaintance rape is sadly very common. Approximately ⅔ of rapes in the United States are committed by someone known to the victim, and even the most well-informed child cannot always protect herself from these dangerous situations. Because of this, it is important to talk to your child about what constitutes date rape before she starts dating. Discuss how rape can happen even with people she is in a relationship with, and how even if she wanted to kiss or touch someone, it is rape if she didn't want to have sex. Let your child know that any escalation of physical touching against someone's will is sexual assault—whether or not he is the quarterback of the football team, her boyfriend, or the boy next door.

While abuse typically happens to girls, it can also impact boys. In fact, more than 2½ million men in the United States have been victims of sexual assault or rape, which means that lessons about inappropriate touch and rape should be shared equally with both genders. In addition to these verbal warnings, young men and women can be empowered to protect themselves through self-defense courses, which you can even take as a family to make less intimidating.

It is also a good idea to use this conversation to stress the importance of always respecting a partner's physical limits. Though partly a stereotype, this is especially important to communicate with boys. Talk to your child about the importance of consent, and emphasize that "no" means no, regardless of how good it feels or how excited a partner seems. Also stress that it is important to get your partner's consent all the way along the sexual continuum. This means checking in with your partner as sexual activity progresses, and always making sure that both of you want to move forward. Teaching your child from an early age to respect a partner—whether sexual or purely romantic—is a gift that will help ensure your child's relationships stay physically and emotionally healthy.

>>> WHAT ARE THE SIGNS OF INAPPROPRIATE SEXUAL CONTACT?

No matter how protective and nurturing you are as a parent, you might come across a situation in which you suspect that your child has been abused in some way. Signs of sexual abuse can include behavioral problems, physical pain, and overtly sexual comments or actions. The following are just possible red flags, and do not mean that abuse has definitely occurred.

• Emotional signs of sexual abuse include sleep problems, depression, withdrawal, seductive behavior or otherwise inappropriate and unusual sexual behavior for your child's age, secretiveness, feelings of low self-worth, and fear or anger at being left somewhere or with someone.

• Physical symptoms of abuse include vaginal or rectal bleeding, pain, itching, swollen genitals, vaginal discharge, and vaginal infections. If your child is young, he may complain of genital pain and irritation, or may engage in compulsive genital touching, even after you have spoken about only touching the private parts in private.

Healing from inappropriate touch

If you discover your child has been abused, try to remain calm. Keep in mind that the extent to which your child can heal after this experience is largely dependent on how the situation is handled. The most important thing you can do for your child is listen. If you try to paint on a happy face after such a serious violation, you will only aggravate the wound. Ask your child about the situation, and stress that it is not her fault and that you are not angry with her. Talking is crucial in the healing process, and your child needs to know that she did nothing wrong, and that she can come talk to you whenever she feels sad, scared, or confused about what happened.

After talking with your child, the first step is to take her for both a medical examination and a psychiatric evaluation. These doctors can also refer you to outside sources in your community that can provide the necessary support and guidance. As you begin the healing process, continually reinforce to your child that the abuse was not her fault and that many people suffer from the same situation. Let her know that she can talk to you about it whenever she wants. It is also important to ensure that your child is removed from any contact with the abuser, and to seek legal retribution as part of the healing process. Taking these concrete, proactive steps will help give your child a sense of resolution and safety.

It is also important to set aside some time to make sure that you are able to cope emotionally. Seek counseling and talk to someone about your feelings. It is not selfish to do so—it is a gift to your child and yourself. Understanding and healing from your own emotional trauma will allow you to process any feelings of anger and guilt, and will enable you to be the best source of comfort and compassion for your child as she heals from this difficult experience.

WHAT TO SAY . . .
IF YOU THINK YOUR CHILD HAS BEEN ABUSED

It can be especially difficult to talk about sexual abuse with a younger child, who may not be able to fully understand what has happened. Try to choose a time and a place in which your child feels very safe, and when you are naturally engaged and talking. Perhaps this is in her car seat, or when you tuck her into bed at night. Make sure you have her attention, and that she is not distracted by anything.

CONVERSATION STARTER: "How have you been feeling lately? Has there been a time when you have felt scared or hurt? You can always tell me about those times."

Give your child a chance to respond, then begin to talk specifically about the genitals and inappropriate touch.

FOLLOW-UP: "Remember that we've talked about how the genitals are your private parts, and how no one should touch you there?"

After opening up the conversation further, wait and listen to your child. Also notice whether she seems uncomfortable or shy. If she doesn't respond, you can ask her more direct questions.

CONVERSATION STARTER: "Has anyone tried to touch your private parts or asked you to touch theirs? Remember that I always want to know if something scary happens, and that you will never be in trouble no matter what you tell me."

If your child acknowledges that she has been touched inappropriately, the most important thing to do is to reassure her that it's not her fault, and give her plenty of time to open up further about what happened.

FOLLOW-UP: "I am so glad you told me about this, and I am so sorry this happened. This is not your fault and we will do everything we can to make sure it never happens again."

Promoting a healthy body image

A healthy body image is the foundation for healthy sexuality and sexual behavior. When boys and girls respect their bodies, they also appreciate the importance of waiting for sex, and of making sex something as special and important as their bodies. Positive self-esteem and body acceptance go further in encouraging children to abstain from casual sex than perhaps any other tool.

The importance of a healthy body image

A healthy body image is an important part of a healthy self-esteem. Research has found that eighty percent of 10-year-old American girls diet in order to lose weight, and that an overwhelming number of young girls aged 11–17 feel such dissatisfaction with their bodies that their number one magic wish is to be thinner. Young boys feel the affects of body image issues as well, though perhaps not to the same degree. Studies show that the number of boys suffering from low self-esteem and low self-worth has grown, as have the rates of depression and suicide among them.

Although we cannot completely control our children's self-esteem, parents play a large role in helping children create and maintain their own feelings of self-worth and pride. Celebrating and caring for the body is a big part of this. It is a good idea to instill these lessons of self-worth from an early age, when young children first begin to understand how their bodies play a part in their lives, and when they first begin to notice that every body is different.

As part of this conversation, you can also stress that even though every person is valuable and every body is uniquely beautiful, weight can sometimes be a health issue. Teach your child that a healthy weight is individual for every person, based on height and build, and that being overly thin is just as unhealthy as being overweight. This shouldn't be a cause of stress for a young child. You can make it fun to be healthy by cooking a variety of interesting foods and encouraging new activities and forms of exercise during playtime.

Setting an example

We often don't realize that what we say around our children is just as important as what we say directly to them. For instance, if you look in the mirror and make disparaging comments or jokes about your own body in front of your child, she will absorb this negative emotion and self-criticism. The same is true when you make comments about the bodies of people around you, even people on television. This negativity is internalized into your child's own mental script, and soon she is in a position to start seeing "fat" on her body, and the bodies of other people.

Body issues are a natural part of the growing up process, and your child will of course have to grapple with these at some point in her life. She will fare much better, however, if she has parents who exhibit healthy pride in their bodies and who promote body acceptance. Your child sees herself as an extension of you, whether she realizes it consciously or not, so when you criticize and find fault with your own body, you are in fact criticizing this smaller

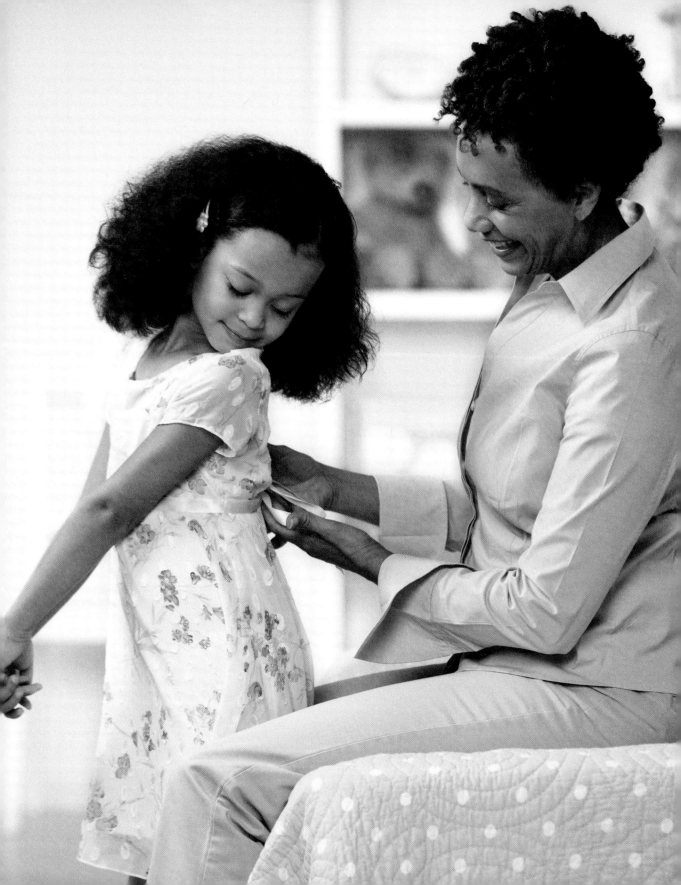

version of your body as well. Actively focus on beginning a dialogue of body acceptance and promoting positive body image and your entire family will reap the rewards of high self-esteem.

The next time you indulge in pizza for dinner, don't leave the table groaning, "I shouldn't have eaten that." Instead, ask your child if she wants to go for a walk to get some exercise, or prepare a healthy meal the next time. This way she will understand the importance of a balanced diet, as well as exercise, without feeling like she did something wrong. Nutritionists agree that piling guilt on food choices makes kids feel like they are bad for choosing unhealthy foods.

Teach your children to look at their bodies not as something to be judged, but as something to be enjoyed and challenged. Take your children rock-climbing at the local gym or hop on bikes for a race around the neighborhood. After you collapse on the lawn post-bike ride, remind your child of this lesson by saying: "Our bodies are so strong, aren't they? Doesn't it feel good to see all the things your body can do?"

Noticing unhealthy eating habits

Children who exhibit unhealthy eating patterns are more likely to develop eating disorders later in adolescence, such as anorexia nervosa and bulimia nervosa. This is why it is so important to note any unhealthy eating patterns that your child exhibits, and make an effort to manage them before they get out of hand.

If you are concerned that your child is developing unhealthy eating habits, you might want to examine the entire family's relationship with food. For example, do you sit down and eat as a family, or do you turn on the television and zone out as you eat? Do you prepare meals together and make cooking part of your nightly routine, or do you make something quick and easy in the microwave? By being more mindful of the way your family eats its meals and encouraging your child to be part of the cooking process, you can truly transform the way he thinks about and experiences food, and can help protect against future problems with eating.

Helping an overweight child

Overeating is also unhealthy and can be a signal that your child is struggling with other issues. Overweight children are much more likely to be overweight adolescents and adults, which can lead to emotional and social difficulty. For your child's well-being, it is important that you treat this problem early. Handle this issue delicately, so that your child doesn't feel punished for the amount of food she eats, or for her body shape.

Make healthy eating the goal of the entire family, and not something that is specific to your child. Make sure that she knows her body is beautiful no matter what shape or size, but that healthy eating and exercise will help her to grow healthy and strong and live a long life (also see page 52).

>>> **YOUR CHILD MAY HAVE AN UNHEALTHY RELATIONSHIP WITH FOOD IF...**
Your child will naturally have likes and dislikes when it comes to food, but she should still enjoy healthy snacks, and the act of sitting down and having a meal should not be painful or unpleasant. Signs that this may be a problem include:
- Finding meals unpleasant, or a source of discomfort or displeasure
- Struggling with eating or with the amount of food to be eaten
- Eating very slowly, or being a very picky eater

Encouraging healthy genital self-image

Healthy genital self-image translates into a healthy sexuality. If your child feels like his genitals are beautiful, healthy, and normal, as opposed to dirty, smelly, or too small—any of the common insecurities or messages that people internalize about their genitals—he will be more likely to treat his body as something precious and valuable. This also means that he will be more likely to respect his body by abstaining from harmful substances or activities, and possibly even more likely to postpone sex. You can incorporate these positive messages every time you talk about anatomy.

Try saying something such as "Your penis is a beautiful and special part of your body," regularly, starting from a young age. Reiterate this to your child during later talks.

It is especially important to instill a healthy genital self-image during adolescence, as children are growing into their bodies for the first time and learning how to adjust to changes in appearance. Young girls are often concerned about the size of their breasts, and may be taunted at school, either for developing at a young age or for developing more slowly than their peers. Young boys might be insecure about the size and shape of their penis and testicles, and might compare their genitals to those of classmates in the locker room. You can help your child develop a healthy genital image by stating that everybody develops at a different rate, and that his body is unique and beautiful.

Take special care to ensure that your daughter is comfortable with her genitals—this does not come as naturally for girls as it does for boys. Don't teach her that her vulva is "dirty" or "bad" by telling her not to wash herself with her hands, or to use a separate washcloth for this part of her body. Instead, encourage her to believe that her genitals are a natural, useful, and beautiful part of her body.

TEACHABLE MOMENT
TALKING ABOUT WEIGHT

Between the ages of 2 and 3, children will begin to notice other people's weight, and may begin to make comments such as: "Daddy, look at that fat woman!" or "Mommy, why is that man so big?" These questions spring naturally to your child's mind when he begins to conceptualize the human body as something to notice, comment on, and even critique.

• **LUCKILY, THESE EARLY** and sometimes embarrassing faux pas can be used to instill not only social grace in your child, but also positive body image. After your child makes a comment or an inquiry about someone's weight or appearance or disability, you can reply by saying: "Every body is built differently. Some mommies are tall, some are short, some are hard, and some are really soft. It is just like how you and your [insert name of friend/brother/classmate] look differently. If we all looked alike, that would be pretty boring, right?" Once you demystify the fact that some people weigh more than others, and that every body is shaped differently, your child should start to understand that not everyone fits into a certain weight range or body type. He will then be more likely to grow up to value his own body and the bodies of others.

CONVERSATION STARTER 1: "Do you notice how your friends all have different body types? Their parents do, too. Part of the reason we all look different is because of our family genetics."

CONVERSATION STARTER 2: "Your friend's daddy is much bigger than yours, isn't he? He is like a football player! Your daddy is tall, which is why he likes to play basketball. Every body is built for something different."

Teaching about conception and birth

Between the ages of 5 and 9, your child will begin to ask questions about what sex means and how babies are made, and you can give honest information about the basic mechanics of sex. Remember that until children hit puberty, they don't conceptualize sex as an erotic act. Younger children simply see it as a geometry puzzle of point A intersecting with point B.

Starting the conversation

For many parents, there is nothing scarier than the question: "Where do babies come from?" This query has caused so much alarm for so many centuries that parents even went to the trouble of creating an elaborate story about a stork delivering babies. As endearing as the stork story is, covering up the truth about conception and birth can create mistrust and apprehension surrounding this crucial sex education lesson. Children are much more observant than adults generally expect, and they start to observe clues about sex at a young age. If you complicate or confuse their early understanding of birth, your child may lose trust in you, and also may grow up with the idea that there is something wrong with talking about sex.

On a very introductory level, you can begin having a conversation about conception and birth as soon as your child becomes curious. Of course, a young child will not understand the realities of sex on an adult level, but there are ways to honestly answer your child's questions about pregnancy and birth without sharing details that you feel are overwhelming or erotic.

As you start to explain the process of conception or birth, you can also insert your own family values and religious or moral beliefs. These are just as important as the mechanical facts, and will help personalize the lesson. With older children, wrapping the information in your family's values will also drive home that you are simply providing important health information, not validating or permitting sexual activity.

Where do babies come from?

This is the most common question asked by children between the ages of 1 and 5. Ideally you are already using the appropriate terms for the genitals, so your child will be prepared to understand some of the logistics. Tell your child that mommies have eggs inside them, just like birds have eggs, though much smaller. Explain that you can't see these eggs because they are inside the body. Then say that daddies have special seeds called sperm, and that when mommies and daddies want to have a baby, his sperm fertilizes her egg, and it becomes a baby. Describe how the baby grows inside the mommy's belly in a special place called the uterus until it is big enough to come out.

This should be enough information to clarify the basics of the process. If she asks further questions, such as, "How does the sperm get to the egg?" or "How does the baby get out?" then you can answer each of these questions, but nothing more. Thus, you might say, "The sperm comes out of the daddy's penis and swims to the egg" or "The baby comes out of the mommy's vagina." Be as simple and open as possible.

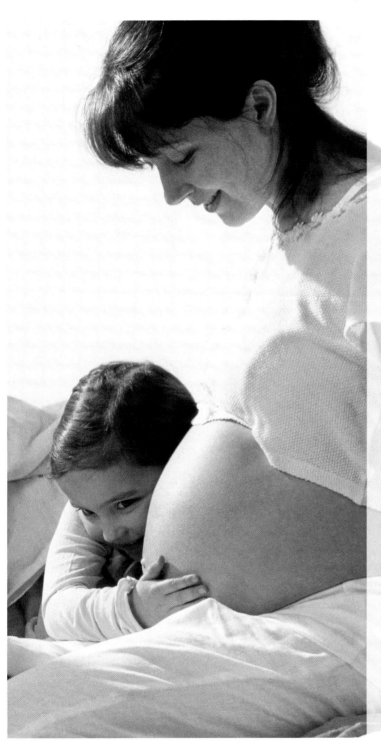

WHAT TO SAY . . .
ABOUT HOW BABIES ARE BORN

....

As your child learns about where babies come from, her next question might be "How are babies born?" The idea of a little person growing inside an adult body and then coming into the world can be a source of endless fascination for children. Giving your child introductory information can help her better understand and come to terms with this miracle of life.

CONVERSATION STARTER: "Babies start out very small. In the first month after they are conceived, they are no bigger than a grain of rice."

Continue talking through a baby's development, in order to set up the birthing process.

FOLLOW-UP: "A baby grows for nine months. Halfway through this time, a baby is 6 inches long, and you can start to see a mommy's tummy grow."

Once your child understands how a baby grows, you can start to talk about the process of labor.

FOLLOW-UP: "Around the end of the nine months, a mommy will start to feel repeating pressure in her tummy. This means that it is almost time for the baby to be born. The process a mommy goes through in order to give birth is called 'labor.'"

If you'd like, you can talk about your own birth choices, such as if you went to the hospital or had a home birth.

FOLLOW-UP: "The mommy begins to push and push until the baby comes out of her vagina."

You can insert your personal values into these conversations. Tell your child that mommies and daddies only create a baby "when they are married," or "when they are in love."

If your child asks a question that you aren't prepared to answer, say something like, "That's a really important question. I am going to find out more about the answer to that question, and then let you know." Take some time to collect your thoughts and then go back to your child with the truth. A straightforward answer will generally satisfy your child's curiosity. However, if your child has more questions for you or seems to have questions that are unusual for her age, you may want to talk with her about what caused her to think of these questions.

The mechanics of sex

Between the ages of 5 and 9, your child will start to notice more of the happenings around him. He may hear the word "sex" on television, or hear his friends talking about something that raises questions. This is the time when you should start being a bit more elaborate and detailed in your explanations of what happens during conception. Although it might sound overwhelming to talk to a 5-year-old about sex, remember that it is natural for children to ask about this mysterious part of growing up and that answering directly can help make it less of a source of fascination.

You might explain the mechanics of sex by simply saying "When a mommy and daddy want to have a baby, he puts his penis inside her vagina, and sperm comes out. When his sperm is inside of her, it travels to her eggs. This is called sex. When he does this, they can become pregnant and have a baby."

Now is also the time to give some early information on the physical changes that allow you to conceive. With a boy, you can tell him that when he gets older and starts to go through puberty, he will start making sperm. For a girl, tell her that she was born with all her eggs, but when she goes through puberty, her eggs will mature so that they can one day grow into a baby.

Continue reinforcing these lessons to your child between the ages of 9 and 12. During these years, your child may ask more detailed questions about sex, and about kissing and other intimate signs of affection that she sees on TV.

You can repeat earlier lessons and put them in a more personal context by saying something like: "When you are older [married, in love, an adult, insert family value here] you will have sex. But right now I am just telling you about it because I don't want you to be confused or scared if you hear about sex at school or on television."

During this stage, you can also go into more detail about the mechanics of sex, explaining erections, ejaculation, and the insemination process. Use the images and information on pages 38–39 to teach your child when and how these processes occur. When your child is between the ages of 13-15 (or earlier if you think necessary), you can also talk about what to expect during sex, including as it relates to sexual response. You don't have to be too graphic, but you should outline what physical and emotional feelings they might experience.

"It is natural for children to ask about sex, and if you answer with straight, simple, truthful information you will help clarify its meaning."

For example, you might say: "When men and women feel sexual attraction, their genitals become filled with blood. In men, this causes an erection. In women, it causes their clitoris to become enlarged and their vaginal opening to widen. Some women also note that their breasts feel tender. This is nature's way of prepping the body for intercourse.

When you feel this arousal, you may also feel a strong desire to have sex. Remember that you can release these feelings without having intercourse, such as through self-stimulation. These feelings are completely natural and healthy, but you should only explore them with another person when you are [older, married, insert personal values here]."

Pregnancy and birth

When your child starts asking questions about where babies come from, try to find real-life moments that can be used to help illustrate your explanations. These real examples will help him better understand the concept of pregnancy. Answer questions as completely and honestly as possible, being careful not to overwhelm your child with unnecessary information.

If you see a pregnant woman on television or walking down the street, you can ask your child if he knows there is a baby inside her stomach. Or, if he has a pregnant relative who would feel comfortable letting him touch her belly, that is an even better opportunity for him to begin to understand the realities of pregnancy.

HOW TO ANSWER THE FIRST QUESTIONS ABOUT SEX

The key to having comfortable parent-child conversations about sex is to make sure you do not provide too much information. Answer questions simply and directly, just as you would answer questions about other physical concerns, such as growing taller or getting sick. Below are some examples of the most common early questions about sex, and possible ways to answer them.

Q. What is sex?
A. Sex is how mommies and daddies are able to make babies.

Q. Where do babies come from?
A. From inside Mommy's tummy.

Q. How does the baby get there?
A. Mommies have eggs inside their uterus, and daddies have sperm. When a mommy and a daddy want to have a child, their egg and sperm meet and turn into a baby.

Q. What are sperm? What are eggs?
A. Men have sperm inside of their testes. Women have eggs inside of their uterus. When a sperm and an egg meet during sex, a woman can become pregnant.

Q. How does the baby get out?
A. When the baby is big enough and strong enough, he comes out of Mommy through her vagina. Then the parents take the baby home from the hospital and take care of it, just like we did with you.

Q. Can boys have babies too?
A. No, only women can have babies. Men don't have eggs like women do. But they help women become pregnant through their sperm, and after the baby is born they have just as big a role in helping to care for the baby as the mommy does.

LEARNING ABOUT REPRODUCTION

Children are fascinated by reproduction. Seeing babies and young animals around them sparks their natural curiosity about where they come from. You can begin teaching them about the reproductive process between the ages of 6 and 8. Keep the information basic and don't overload your child with detail. Try to maintain the exchange as a dialogue and approach it in a light-hearted way so that you keep your young audience engaged. It will help to have several conversations about this topic, rather than just one.

AFTER THIS LESSON YOUR CHILD WILL BE MORE LIKELY TO...
- Understand the mechanics of sex, including what a penis is for and why it changes shape
- Know how an egg is fertilized, what an embryo is, and how an embryo develops into a fetus
- Appreciate how a baby grows and develops inside the uterus
- Feel comfortable asking you questions on the reproductive process
- Be better informed and less overwhelmed by big questions, like "Where did I come from?" and "How are babies made?".

1   WHAT IS SPERM AND HOW IS IT MADE?

A sperm is a very tiny male reproductive cell. It is made up of three parts and looks a bit like a tadpole. It has a relatively large head, which contains all the genetic material needed to make a baby; a body or midpiece, which gives it energy; and a long tail, which helps it to swim. Sperm is made in the testes—it takes about 72 days for one sperm to grow! To stay healthy, sperm need to be kept at a constant temperature that is three to five degrees below body temperature. The scrotum (the sack that holds the testes) has a built-in thermostat, which keeps sperm at the right temperature while they are being stored. Each time a man ejaculates, he releases approximately 200-500 million sperm cells. An adult male will then continue recreating sperm thoughout his life.

FLACCID PENIS   **ERECT PENIS**

2   WHY DOES A PENIS BECOME ERECT?

Explain to your child that a man's penis, which is normally soft and hangs down, can grow bigger and harder when the spongy tissue inside the penis fills with blood. It then becomes longer and wider and sticks outward and upward from the body. Sometimes an erection happens for no obvious reason—maybe in the morning when he first wakes up, or when he is having thoughts that make him feel good. Or he may get an erecton when he is having intercourse. In this case, the man fits his erect penis into the woman's vagina and they have sex until the sperm come out and start to swim up to her egg.

1. FERTILIZATION OF THE EGG

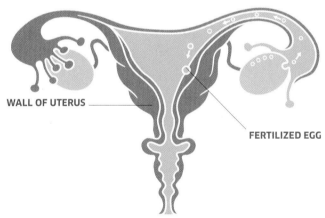

FALLOPIAN TUBE

UTERUS

CERVIX

VAGINA

OVARY

RELEASED EGGS
FROM THE OVARY

SPERM SWIMS UP THE
FALLOPIAN TUBE

2. ATTACHMENT OF THE EMBRYO

WALL OF UTERUS

FERTILIZED EGG

BABY IN UTERO: 16 WEEKS

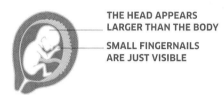

THE HEAD APPEARS
LARGER THAN THE BODY

SMALL FINGERNAILS
ARE JUST VISIBLE

BABY IN UTERO: 32 WEEKS

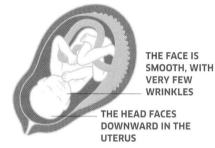

THE FACE IS
SMOOTH, WITH
VERY FEW
WRINKLES

THE HEAD FACES
DOWNWARD IN THE
UTERUS

BABY IN UTERO: 40 WEEKS

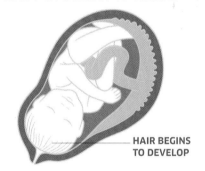

HAIR BEGINS
TO DEVELOP

3   WHAT HAPPENS WHEN A SPERM MEETS THE EGG?

Explain that sperm are excellent swimmers. They swim through the cervix, into the uterus, then into the fallopian tubes. If an egg is there, hundreds of sperm swim to meet it. The first to penetrate it is the one that makes a baby. Next, the fertilized egg moves down the fallopian tube and starts to grow. Around the third day after fertilization, the egg has become 64 separate cells. When it reaches the uterus, the egg attaches to the thick lining that's been building there over the course of the month. It is no longer an egg, but an embryo—which is too small to see, but is the start of a baby.

4   HOW DOES A BABY GROW?

It takes about nine months for a baby to develop. After eight weeks, the baby isn't called an embryo any more, but a fetus. By 12 weeks, it has arms, legs, fingers and toes, and a face. By 24 weeks, the bones start to harden and the fetus can hear sounds. Explain that the baby continues to grow until it is about 36 weeks old, when it generally settles into a head-down position. This means it is nearly ready to be born.

Learning together

Puberty and physical changes

Puberty can be both a time of exciting growth and difficult change. The more you prepare your child for these changes, the easier this transition will be. Your child will not feel as out of place or frightened by puberty if he knows that these changes are normal, that they happen to everyone, and that emotions are welcome and can be discussed openly and honestly.

Starting the conversation

It is a good idea to begin discussing puberty well before your child enters this period, ideally around the age of 7 or 8. Girls are reaching puberty much earlier than in previous generations, sometimes as early as 9 years old. We don't know why this is: one theory is the use of insecticides, which breaks down into compounds that may affect estrogen levels in young girls. Other theories revolve around hormones in our food and a higher fat, less active lifestyle.

This means the discussion needs to start sooner than you might previously have planned. And, if young girls are heading into puberty, young boys need the talk as well. Their physical changes might not reflect puberty as early as girls, but the mental and emotional changes will certainly start earlier, thanks to both hormones and the changing bodies of those around him.

What is puberty?

Puberty is the blanket term used for all the physical and emotional changes that occur during adolescence. During puberty, the body goes through growth and development more rapidly than at any other time of a person's life, except infancy. This is why pre-teens and teens often feel tired and irritable—their bodies are growing rapidly due to changing hormones.

The processes of puberty begin in both boys and girls when the brain releases a gonadotropin-releasing hormone, or GnRH for short. GnRH stimulates the pituitary gland, located at the base of the brain, which in turn stimulates two additional hormones, luteinizing hormone (LH for short) and follicle-stimulating hormone (FSH for short). This generally happens between the ages of 9 and 16 in girls, and between the ages of 10 and 15 in boys.

However, it is important to share with your child that everyone hits puberty at different times, and that different stages of puberty occur at different times. In other words, a boy might begin to grow pubic hair at the age of 10, but might not have a nocturnal emission, or ejaculate in his sleep, until years later. Alternately, a girl might get her first period at the age of 10, but not see her breasts develop until much later. Reassure your child that different paces of development are completely normal and healthy. It is also a good idea to schedule a physical check-up at least once a year, so that your child's doctor can check development and offer similar reassurance.

When puberty does officially begin, the hormones act upon boys and girls differently. In girls, the follicle-stimulating hormone and the luteinizing hormone stimulate the ovaries, creating estrogen. In boys, FSH and LH travel to the testicles, where they signal the production of sperm and testosterone.

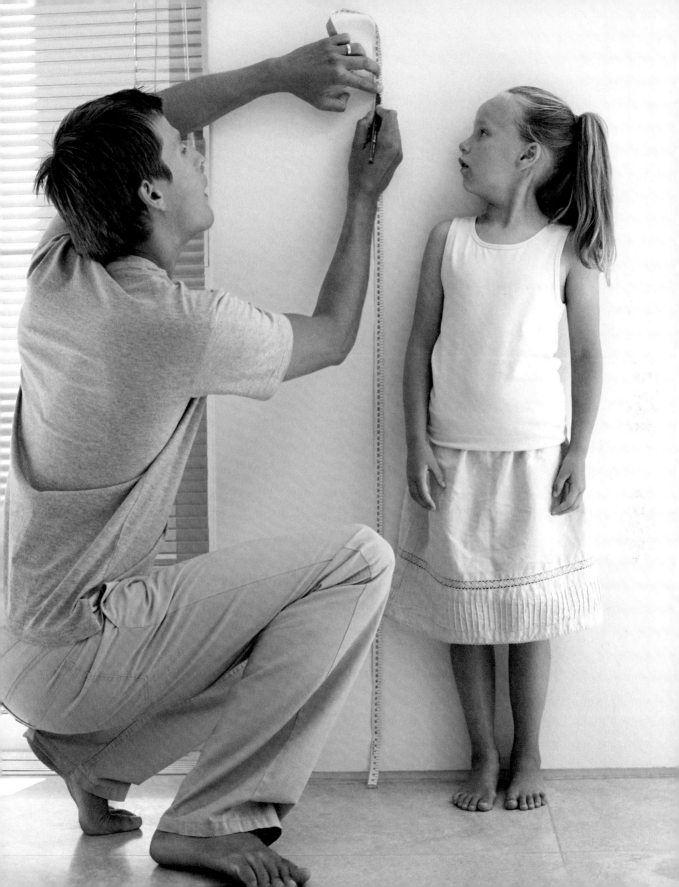

Physical changes of puberty

Though puberty generally begins slightly earlier for girls, the general stages of growth are similar for both genders. First, limbs begin to widen and lengthen; next, genitals begin to mature; finally, hair growth and further physical changes transform your child's body into that of an adult.

8–11 years old. Boys and girls might begin to experience a bit of a growth spurt, and their legs and arms get longer. Boys' shoulders widen, their testicles begin to mature, and testosterone production begins. In girls, ovaries begin to enlarge and hormone production also begins. Some girls get their first period during this time.

11–13 years old. Girls and boys continue to experience a growth spurt, including height increase and weight gain. Acne generally develops around this time as well, as does

SEXPLANATION
WHAT ARE NOCTURNAL EMISSIONS?

Also referred to as spontaneous orgasm, nocturnal emissions are the involuntary release of semen during sleep. These generally begin during the early stages of puberty in order to release excess sperm as sperm production begins. Nocturnal emissions can occur due to sexual dreams or thoughts, but this is not always the case.

Using the correct medical term, "nocturnal emissions," will help normalize and justify the experience and make it what it is—a common and completely typical and natural part of growing up. Explain that many adult men still experience nocturnal emissions from time to time. You can also mention to your child that he might hear these called wet dreams from his peers or on television, and that these terms mean the same thing.

a stronger body odor. This body odor is a result of the new hormones, which affect glands in the skin that create malodorous chemicals.

Girls will gain weight around their hips, and they will begin to develop breast buds, if they have not done so already. Their nipple size may also change, and they may experience soreness around their nipples and breasts. It is common for breasts to develop at different rates, so that one breast might actually be larger than the other. Reassure your daughter that this is normal and that it may change over time—although you can also point out that it is not uncommon for adult women to have some slight difference in size between their left and right breasts.

In boys, the penis will begin to enlarge, both in length and width, and the testicles will grow larger. Pubic hair, underarm hair, and chest hair might also begin to develop, though sparingly and fine at first. Later, it may grow in more completely and with more coarseness.

13–15 years old. Your child's growth spurt continues. Boys commonly experience their first erection from a sexual thought, and perhaps their first ejaculation, though this may happen earlier. Nocturnal emissions (a.k.a. "wet dreams") might also begin to occur. Boys' voices begin to deepen and perhaps crack. Facial hair also begins to grow, though sparingly at first.

In girls, the vagina begins to enlarge and may also begin to produce a clear or white discharge. This is a normal part of the self-cleaning process of the female genitals, and is not a cause for concern, provided there are no other symptoms that accompany it. Most girls tend to have their first period during this time. Initial periods can be very erratic, so your daughter might have her first period, but then not experience another one for several months. You can reassure your daughter that this initial menstrual irregularity is not a cause for concern, but it is still a good idea to begin regular ob/gyn appointments after her

TEACHABLE MOMENTS
TALKING ABOUT MENSTRUATION

A good time to begin talking about menstruation is when your child is 8 or 9 years old. This is true for both boys and girls—each child should know about this key part of growing up. Menstruation can be one of the scariest parts of puberty, so look for natural teachable moments when you can explain this process in a relaxed way.

• **WATCHING TELEVISION:** An easy time to start a conversation about menstruation is while watching television. When you see a commercial for tampons or menstrual pads, ask your daughter if she knows what the commercial is about, then respond with an explanation about what it means to have your period. Let her know that some girls reach puberty sooner than others, and say something like **"It might be years before you have your period, but I want you to have all the information you need now, so that you won't be scared or confused the first time it happens."** You can use this same moment to talk to your son about menstruation, letting him know when and how this may impact the girls in his class.

• **AT THE STORE:** Use the female hygiene aisle to begin a conversation about the different ways women manage menstruation. For example, you might say **"I like to use tampons when I am on my period, just because I find that to be most comfortable. But when you start getting your period, you might want to use menstrual pads [point to pads on shelf]."** You can then ask your daughter if she is nervous about getting her period, or if she knows anyone that has already begun menstruating.

• **WITH AN OLDER SIBLING:** If you have an older daughter that has already begun menstruating, you might share her experiences with your younger child. This can help normalize the process. Try saying something such as, **"Your sister isn't feeling well today because she is on her period. Do you know what that means?"**

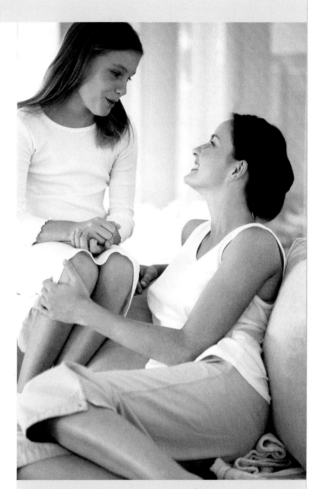

CONVERSATION STARTER 1: "Do you know how a tampon works, and how a pad works? They are very different, but they both work to absorb your period and are easy and discreet methods of feminine protection."

CONVERSATION STARTER 2: "Have any of your friends started to get their period yet? Do you talk about it with them? What do they say about the experience?"

first period, so that she can learn more about maintaining good sexual health from a trusted medical professional.

15–19 years old. Boys sometimes reach their adult height when they are 16 or 17 years old, while others may continue growing until the age of 21. By this age, the penis and testicles have reached their adult size, and body hair and facial hair grows in completely. The voice deepens to its adult timbre.

Girls generally reach their adult height when they are 15 or 16 years old. Breasts reach their adult size around the age of 15, and pubic hair growth is also complete. Menstruation becomes regular and monthly.

The menstrual cycle

A good time to begin discussing menstruation is around the age of 9 years old, since more young girls are reaching puberty at this age. Bring up this topic at the same time for boys and girls, as it is important for boys to know and understand what menstruation is as well, and how this relates to conception and birth.

Explain that as a girl reaches adolescence she starts to go through a monthly menstrual cycle, when the lining of her uterus will shed. Each month her body releases hormones that create an amazing process that will one day allow her to get pregnant [inserting your personal value about sex and pregnancy here]. You can also explain what happens during each of the four stages of the menstrual cycle: the pre-ovulatory phase, the ovulation phase, the post-ovulatory phase and the menstrual phase, using the chart and the definitions on pages 48–49.

The realities of menstruation

You can help your daughter feel comfortable with the idea of menstruation by explaining that it is a gift that means she can one day have children. It is a good idea to also mention that many women experience cramping during menstruation. Explain that this occurs when the uterus contracts, which happens in order to help the lining of the uterus shed. Cramps vary in intensity, and pain relievers like acetametaphin and motrin, or natural remedies like applying heat, are helpful in relieving the symptom. **Minimize any fears your child may have** about menstrual pain by saying something such as: "Some women do experience cramps or other symptoms every month. But there are remedies to help treat this pain, and most women find one that makes their period comfortable and usually not even very noticeable."

Choosing feminine protection

Many young girls are nervous about using feminine protection for the first time. Your daughter may worry that kids at school will be able to see that she is using feminine products, especially if she uses bulky menstrual pads. Tampons can be worrisome as well because they are more difficult to use, and can be uncomfortable if not inserted properly. Some

"Help your daughter feel comfortable with the idea of menstruation by explaining that it is a gift that means she can one day have children."

SEXPLANATION
WHAT ARE THE TYPES OF FEMININE PROTECTION?

To help your daughter choose which type of protection she is most comfortable with, explain the benefits and complications of using menstrual pads, tampons, and menstrual cups, then let her experiment with each. Reassure your child that when used properly, all options are comfortable, discreet, and safe. Choosing the right one for your body is simply a matter of personal preference.

TYPE OF PROTECTION	PROS AND CONS
TAMPONS Tampons are inserted into the vagina and absorb the menstrual flow from inside your body. They come in multiple absorbencies, so you can choose your tampon based on how much you are bleeding. Tampons allow you to swim, play sports, and keep your normal routine.	**PROS:** When inserted properly, tampons can be easier and more comfortable than pads. **CONS:** When not inserted correctly, tampons can be uncomfortable. In rare cases, they can lead to Toxic Shock Syndrome, a bacterial infection that occurs when a tampon is left in too long.
MENSTRUAL PADS Menstrual pads are disposable and are worn inside the underwear. Pads come in all different shapes and sizes to fit different needs and levels of blood flow.	**PROS:** Menstrual pads are easy to use, especially when first getting used to feminine protection. **CONS:** Pads can be messy or uncomfortable, and they can be difficult to use when playing sports.
MENSTRUAL CUPS Used less commonly than tampons or pads, menstrual cups are inserted inside the vagina to "catch" the menstrual flow. Worn a few inches below the cervix, they can be used for up to 6 to 12 hours, and they come in a variety of materials (rubber, silicone, etc.).	**PROS:** Menstrual cups are healthy, safe, environmentally-friendly, and cost effective, since you can reuse one cup for many years. **CONS:** They can be difficult to insert and remove, particularly at first, and some women find them to be too large or uncomfortable.

girls also worry that tampons can be "lost" inside the body. To assuage these fears, refer back to the female anatomy diagram on pages 24–25, and explain how it is impossible for a tampon to escape beyond the cervix.

Some parents feel hesitant about young girls using tampons. Some even wonder if inserting a tampon into the vagina compromises their daughter's virginity. A girl's hymen can be broken by playing sports or in other physical activities. However, virginity is about the act of sex and the emotional ground that is crossed, and this cannot be compromised by using a tampon. Tampons are a safe and hygienic way for women to manage menstruation, and many tampon companies are now making slim fit tampons specifically for young girls. If your daughter does decide to use tampons, remember to explain that she needs to change her tampon every 4-6 hours in order to prevent Toxic Shock Syndrome, a rare but potentially fatal disease caused by the presence of a bacterial toxin.

Show your child how a tampon works to absorb her period without leaks by placing the tampon in a glass of water and watching it expand to absorb the "menstrual flow." Explain that this exact process can occur inside her body.

Learning together

LEARNING ABOUT MENSTRUATION

For a girl, starting her periods can be a scary change. Talk your child through the phases of the menstrual cycle as early as age 7 or 8, so that she understands what will happen inside her body. During this time, you can also address practicalities such as choosing feminine protection. Boys should also learn about the menstrual cycle, both because it has implications for them, too, and because it will help them overcome any squeamishness about the subject.

AFTER THIS LESSON YOUR CHILD WILL BE MORE LIKELY TO...

- Be prepared for her first menstrual cycle so that the experience will be a positive one
- Understand that menstrual bleeding is a very normal process and that she doesn't need to feel embarrassed or worried about it
- Appreciate what is happening inside her body each month and why
- Know which type of protection she wishes to try and how to use it
- Be more willing to talk to you about any questions or problems she has
- Have an understanding (if your child is a boy) of what girls experience.

---

1 WHAT IS THE MENSTRUAL CYCLE?

Explain to your child that the menstrual cycle begins on the first day of menstruation and ends on the day before the next period starts. The average length of the menstrual cycle is 28 days, although it can be as short as 21 days or as long as 40 days—all are normal. The cycle may be unpredictable when your child first starts menstruating. It will usually settle into a more regular pattern within the first year. The cycle has four phases (see page 47), which are controlled by hormones.

2 WHAT IS OVULATION?

Show your child the diagrams on the next page and explain how every month, about 20 tiny eggs start to grow in one of the ovaries. Usually, one egg grows bigger than the others and is released into the fallopian tube, which connects the ovary to the uterus. This generally happens about 10–16 days before the start of menstruation. If the egg is not fertilized, it is absorbed back into the body. At this time, the uterus lining breaks up and is released through the vagina as a period.

3 HOW DO YOU USE A TAMPON?

Use the information on p. 45 to ensure your child is aware of the different types of feminine protection available. The most difficult of these to learn to use is the tampon, though in many ways it is also the most convenient and comfortable. Your child will probably be nervous about using a tampon for the first time, so it is a good idea to walk her through the diagrams at right to make sure she knows how to insert it. To start, she may want to choose the smallest size of tampon, as these are often the most comfortable. Explain that she will need to sit or stand in a relaxed position—it may help to place one leg on the toilet seat or bathtub. Next, she holds the middle of the tampon, where the smaller inner tube meets the larger one, with the string pointing downward. She gently pushes the outer applicator into the vagina until it is completely inside, then pushes the inner tube up inside the outer one to release the absorbent tampon. She can use her thumb and middle finger to remove the applicator, making sure that the string hangs outside the vaginal opening. Reassure your child that this process is easy to learn with just a bit of practice.

1 PRE-OVULATORY PHASE

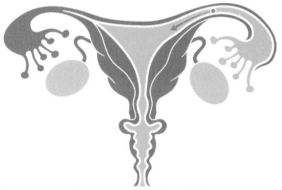

FALLOPIAN TUBE

OVARY

UTERINE CAVITY

OVUM (EGG)

VAGINA

Large amounts of follicle stimulating hormone and small amounts of luteinizing hormone are produced. Estrogen increases and the uterine lining thickens.

2 OVULATION PHASE

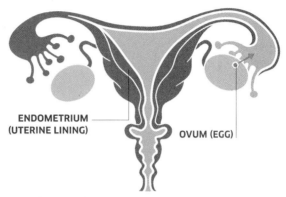

ENDOMETRIUM (UTERINE LINING)

OVUM (EGG)

Increased levels of estrogen decrease FSH production. The egg is released, which is followed by a release of the hormone progesterone.

3 POST-OVULATORY PHASE 3

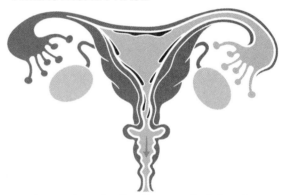

Progesterone increases. The lining of the uterus continues to thicken and, if conception has occurred, it will now be ready to sustain the fertilized egg.

4 MENSTRUAL PHASE

If an egg has not been fertilized by now, the lining of the uterus is shed and the menstrual flow begins. When the flow ends, the pre-ovulatory phase begins again.

INSERTING A TAMPON

Show your child how her body is created to fit a tampon easily and painlessly. The first step at right shows how to slide the applicator inside the outer tube of the tampon, for easy insertion (see full instruction at right). The second step shows how to remove the applicator, leaving the tampon secure inside the body.

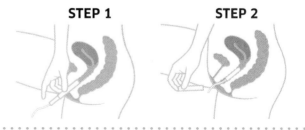

STEP 1   STEP 2

Learning together

Learning together

LEARNING ABOUT PUBERTY

To help your child negotiate puberty successfully, try to fully prepare him for the physical and emotional changes that lie ahead. Around the age of 9 or 10, let him know that acne, growth spurts, and weight gain are all normal during this time. Explain that it makes no difference when you start your sexual development. It doesn't affect what someone will be like as an adult. Boys and girls should see and learn about both sets of diagrams so they learn how changes impact both sexes.

AFTER THIS LESSON YOUR CHILD WILL BE MORE LIKELY TO...
- Take the first signs of puberty in his stride when he begins to experience these changes
- Have a greater understanding of what friends may be going through if they are going through puberty earlier
- Maintain a healthy body image as he moves into adulthood
- Feel that he can approach you for help if he doesn't understand how his body is changing
- Realize that everyone has to deal with similar adolescent challenges and there's nothing to feel embarrassed about or ashamed of.

1 HOW DO HORMONES IMPACT MY BODY DURING PUBERTY?

Does your child know what hormones are? Explain that hormones act like messengers, traveling around the body and coordinating difficult processes, such as how you grow and how you digest your food. Tell your child that some time after the age of 9 (and perhaps as late as 15), his brain will release gonadotropin-releasing hormone (GnRH), which stimulates the production of two more hormones called luteinizing hormone (LH) and follicle stimulating hormone (FSH). In boys, these two hormones trigger the body to produce testosterone. In girls, these hormones stimulate the ovaries to produce estrogen and progesterone. Tell your child that estrogen, progesterone, and testosterone are known as the sex hormones. These sex hormones (depending on the sex of your child) are responsible for the bodily changes that turn children into adults.

2 WILL HORMONES CAUSE ME TO GAIN ADDITIONAL WEIGHT?

This can be a common concern, especially for girls. Your child may worry if he is gaining too much weight or too little, depending on how his body develops compared to his peers' bodies. Explain to your child that boys and girls do start to fill out when they go through puberty, and that boys in particular develop more muscle mass. This is perfectly normal and an important part of growing into a sexually mature adult. Also explain that it may take three or four years in order to gain all the weight and muscle mass you will have as an adult—and that even after puberty, these can continue to change.

3 WHY DO I SMELL DIFFERENTLY?

Changing hormones have a big impact on personal scent, which can be strange or even worrisome for children. Explain that during puberty, your hormones are working overtime and this causes you to sweat more than you ever have before and in places where you might not have had sweat before. Sometimes this sweat or wetness can be smelly and create body odor (BO). Reassure your child that bathing or showering more frequently can help combat body odor. It is a good idea to introduce your child to deodorant at this age, which can help him feel more secure about these hormonal changes and more comfortable about participating in sports or other active hobbies.

4   WHAT HAPPENS TO GIRLS DURING PUBERTY?

Ask your child to identify some changes that girls experience during puberty. Use the diagrams at right to help describe these changes. If he has trouble beginning, point out how a girl changes shape as she grows, becoming taller and heavier. Show how her breasts become bigger and fuller, her hips become more rounded, and how hair grows in the armpits and around the genitals. Explain that inside a girl's body, her reproductive organs are also developing. As her ovaries begin to release eggs, she starts to menstruate. In addition, her skin may become oilier and she may develop pimples. Explain that a girl's body continues growing until her breasts are grown, her body hair is at its adult thickness, and she reaches her adult height (diagram at far right).

ADOLESCENT GIRL

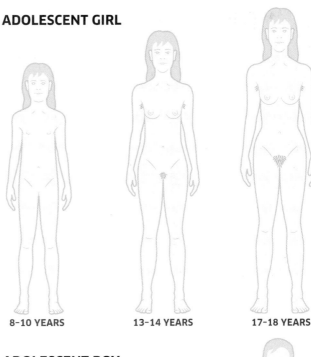

8-10 YEARS   13-14 YEARS   17-18 YEARS

5   WHAT HAPPENS TO BOYS DURING PUBERTY?

Ask your child to identify the changes that boys undergo during puberty. To start, he can look at the diagrams and point out things that he already knows about, such as weight gain or hair growth. Explain that a boy's shoulders will broaden, he will become more muscular, grow taller, and hair will begin to grow in his armpits and around the genitals, though it may be quite fine at first. The penis and testicles also get bigger. Next, body hair becomes thicker and grows on the arms, legs, face, and chest, and thickens on the genitals. A boy's voice will deepen, or "crack," and he will begin to sweat more. His skin also becomes oilier, which means he may get pimples. The diagram at far right shows the boy grown to his adult height and size.

ADOLESCENT BOY

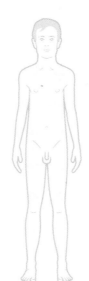
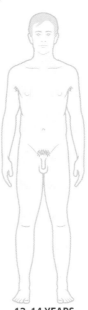
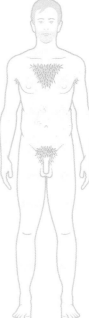

8-10 YEARS   13-14 YEARS   17-18 YEARS

Learning together

Pleasuring and self-stimulation

Part of helping your child feel comfortable with his growing sexual thoughts and feelings is discussing the act of self-pleasuring. This can be a difficult topic to come to terms with as a parent, but discussing self-stimulation is a way of normalizing sexual feelings, and of helping your child find a safe way to release these.

Talking about self-touch

Around age 9, you can begin talking about self-stimulation, just as you originally began talking about touching of the genitals when your child was a toddler. This means that as you teach your daughter about her sexual anatomy and the changes that come with adolescence, you also teach her that it is healthy and normal to look at and explore her genitals. Show her the clitoris on a diagram (see page 25) and tell her that this is an area rich in nerve endings, which means there will be a lot of sensation there. Tell her that it is normal to explore this area and to see how it feels now and as she gets older. Do the same for your son, showing him a diagram of the penis and testes (see page 24).

Around age 12, you might say: "As you start to get older, your hormones might cause you to have some sexual feelings. That's completely normal and it is happening for everyone else in your grade, too." Explain openly that you expect she'll have some thoughts about sex and that this is normal.

Simply by letting your child know that you understand and accept her natural progression into a sexual human being, you can help her to feel safe coming to you with sexual questions. This is very important. By establishing yourself as someone your child can come to for information and support about sexual questions and concerns, you are helping to ensure that you are one of the most dominant influences in establishing your child's sexual knowledge, and in guiding her through the sexual decision-making process. This means that your child will be less likely to get the majority of her information and guidance from media influences or from her peers.

It is especially important that you address the topic of sexual pleasure with young girls, as it is common to sometimes brush over the reality of sexual urges in girls and women. If you instead let your daughter know that her feelings are natural and normal, she will be less likely to feel ashamed or embarrassed of her sexuality. She will also be more likely to feel in control of her sexuality, which means that there will be fewer reasons for her to succumb to peer pressure or the temptation to have sex.

Talking about masturbation

Around this same age, you may get more specific about using masturbation as a form of sexual release. This can be a cringe-worthy topic for parents, but remember that it can mean the difference between whether your child chooses to delay intercourse or not. Having this conversation allows you to suggest other ways for your teenager to manage strong sexual feelings, rather than jumping into sexual activity before being mentally or emotionally prepared for it. When you teach your child to harness his own sexual feelings and understand and own them for himself, he is much less likely to be tempted by peer pressure or get carried away in sexual situations with someone else, and thus much more likely to wait to have sex.

To begin with, it might help if you use the term "self-stimulation" instead of masturbation—this will probably be easier for you to say and for your child to hear. Talk to your child about how self-stimulating is a healthy way to experience sexual pleasure, and how it can protect him from both emotional pain and physical risks such as sexually transmitted diseases and pregnancy. While your child might appear to not to be paying attention—and might act embarrassed or outraged by rolling his eyes and groaning throughout the talk—rest assured that he is listening to everything that you are saying, and that you are taking a serious step to protect him from unsafe sex.

Stimulation with vibrators

While most teenage boys have no trouble figuring out self-stimulation and accomplishing orgasms, it can be much more difficult for girls. Adolescent girls often have a hard time figuring out how to self-stimulate, and thus can't be easily empowered to discover and achieve their own sexual pleasure. Talking openly about self-stimulation can help your daughter feel comfortable exploring this, but it may also help to provide some more practical assistance. **Parents of girls 15 or 16 years old or older** might want to consider buying their daughters a small, clitoral vibrator to help them become acquainted with their own anatomy and sexual pleasure. It doesn't need to be anything big or scary, or anything that requires vaginal insertion. It is just a small tool to help your daughter learn about her body and her sexual pleasure without engaging in any emotionally or physically dangerous behaviors.

WHAT TO SAY . . .
TALKING ABOUT SELF-STIMULATION

Many parents feel that self-stimulation is not a topic they should discuss with their child, but the reality is that it can make a huge difference in the way your child feels about his body, and in how long he waits to become sexually active. Try to broach this topic sensitively.

CONVERSATION STARTER: "I know that your hormones have you thinking about sex a lot, and that you are curious about experimenting with these thoughts. These feelings are a normal part of being an adult, but even though your body is ready for sex, your mind isn't."

Your child may be looking embarrassed by this point, but continue on. Even if he is avoiding eye contact or rolling his eyes, you would be surprised how much he is taking in.

FOLLOW-UP: "You still have plenty of developing to do and I wouldn't want you to rush into sex before you are ready and get hurt. Sex feels good, but there are other ways to get that good feeling without rushing into sex with another person."

It is important to acknowledge the temptation of pleasure. By denying the existence of this natural motivation to experience sexual pleasure, you might cause your child to feel he must act out these feelings secretively and often unsafely. Being open about these feelings can be a powerful protective measure.

FOLLOW-UP: "I know it is embarrassing to talk about, but touching yourself in and around your genitals is an absolutely normal and healthy way to explore your sexual feelings. A lot of teenagers and adults self-stimulate as a way to release sexual feelings and to get in touch with their bodies and their sexuality. This is true for men and women—nearly everyone self-stimulates, and it is a much better option than engaging in sex with someone before you are ready."

Encouraging a healthy lifestyle

Children that learn to care for and appreciate their bodies and make healthy lifestyle decisions are also much more likely to take care of their bodies as they grow up and are confronted with sexual decisions. Help your child view his body as something to protect and nourish, and he will be better equipped to stay emotionally and physically safe in the future.

Setting nutritional standards

Raising children to make healthy eating choices has never been of more pressing concern. Nearly one-fifth of American 4-year-olds are obese. The health concerns that accompany this excess weight, including diabetes, are present in young children more than ever before. If your child is not exposed to a healthy nutrition program from a young age, she could be at risk for health and weight problems in the near and long-term future. Obese children are more likely to grow up to become obese adults, with all of the physical and emotional hardships associated with obesity. Research also shows that obese parents are more likely to have obese children, so making healthy lifestyle choices for yourself will go a long way in helping your children to make these same healthy choices.

Growing kids have different nutrition requirements throughout each stage of their development. While you should always talk to your doctor about your child's nutritional needs, on average, your child's daily consumption of calories should be 1,300 a day between 1–3 years; 1,800 a day between 4–6 years; and 2,000 a day between 7–10 years. Boys of 11–14 years generally need 2,500 a day, and boys of 15–18 years need 3,000 a day. Girls of 11–14 years generally need 2,200 a day, and girls of 15–18 years need 2,500 a day.

It is a good idea to avoid using food as a reward. It is tempting to reward good behavior with snacks and sweets, yet this can cause your child to have an unhealthy relationship with food. Children who receive sugary rewards start to see healthy foods as punishment, instead of enjoying their taste and associating them with strong, healthy bodies. A better choice is to make toys, activities, or playtime a treat.

Plan to make health and variety the focus of your meals. When preparing meals, don't make lower calories, carbs, or fat grams the focus. Instead, create balanced, varied meals that include all the food groups. Bring in new and seasonal vegetables, like edamame or summer squash, and your child will be much more likely to stay interested and involved in nutrition.

Encouraging athleticism

Study after study has shown the benefit of sports in a young child's life. Sports teach endurance, discipline, confidence, and even positive body image. When your child learns that his body is something of value, strength, and power, he will be less likely to critique himself based on weight and appearance—and more likely to be proud of how his body is capable of performing. In addition, the endorphins released during exercise help promote feel-good chemicals in the brain and positive, happy feelings. Active children are also more likely to maintain a healthy weight in a way that is much more empowering and esteem-building than simply cutting calories.

If your child is not interested in team sports or organized athletics, try to get him moving in a different way. For instance, ask him to walk around the block with you after dinner, or take her to the park for a game of tag. The important thing is to be active for at least 20–30 minutes a day—it doesn't matter if that activity comes in the form of baseball or playing in the leaves.

Teaching healthy sleep habits

Sleep is a crucial part of a healthy lifestyle. Research shows that children ages 1–3 need 12–15 hours of sleep, children ages 3–5 need 11–13 hours, children ages 5–12 need 9–11 hours, and teenagers need 9–10 hours. These numbers might seem extreme, but they are real: sleep affects everything from physical health to cognitive function to mood and weight.

You can help your child develop healthy sleeping habits by putting her to bed and waking her up at the same time every day. Even on the weekends, it is a good idea for her to sleep in no more than an hour later. This will keep your child's body on a regular sleep cycle, which is crucial for healthy sleep behavior.

To help encourage proper sleep habits, it is a good idea for your child prepare for bed at least an hour beforehand. Studies have found that sitting in front of the television and computer can interfere with R.E.M. sleep later in the night due to the flashing lights of the screens. Instead, dim the lights, and have your child read a book or play a board game.

Older children might not choose to follow this routine. If your child chooses to stay awake in her bedroom, it is generally effective to let her make this decision for herself, though you can prohibit cell phone or television and computer use after a certain time. After a few mornings of feeling too tired to get out of bed, she will be more likely to start seeking more rest.

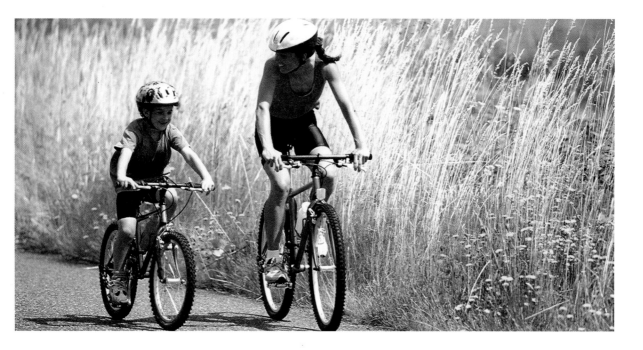

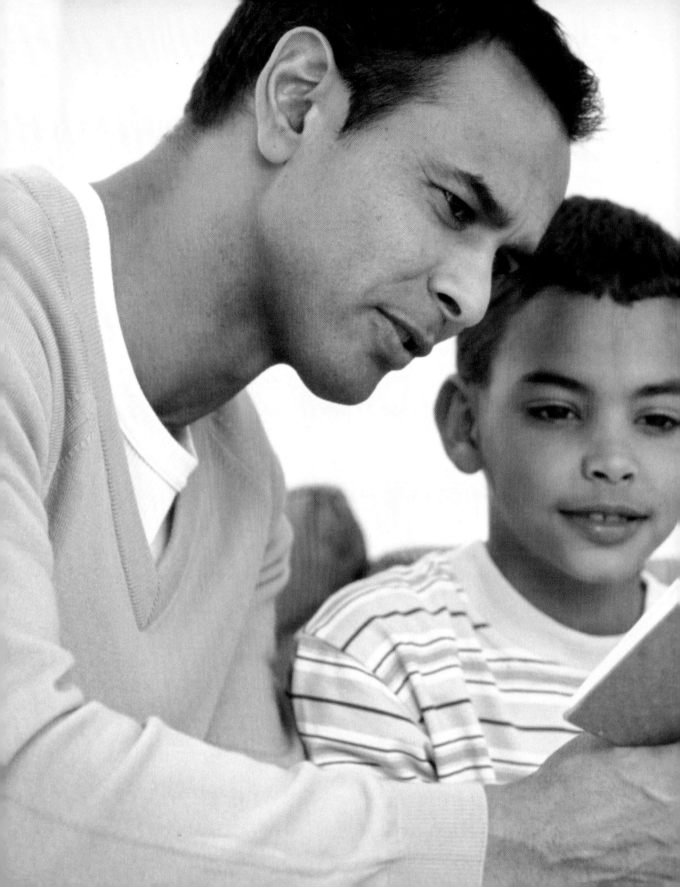

2

TALKING ABOUT THE MIND

ASSESSING YOUR VALUES: THE MIND

The cliché is true—your mind really is your most important sexual organ. The way you think about sexuality will determine how your children think about sex, from infancy all the way through adolescence and into adulthood. Take some time to analyze how you view the emotional impact of sex, sexual orientation, and sexual decision-making. Answer these questions privately, then discuss with your partner what values you want to pass along to your child.

EXPLORING SEXUAL THOUGHT

Think about the sexual values you grew up with, and about if and how you want to pass the same values on to your child.

• What lessons did your parents teach you about sex and sexuality, verbally or nonverbally?

• What moral guidelines help direct your own sexual decisions?

• What do you remember about your sexual thoughts as a teenager?

• How do your religious or moral beliefs and thoughts impact your views about the appropriate time to become sexually active?

• What do you think are the benefits of waiting until adulthood to have sex?

• What do you think it means to have "responsible" sex? How does planning your sexual experiences encourage this?

EXPLORING EMOTIONS

Consider the emotional history of your sexual relationships. This will impact all of your early lessons about sex, although you won't discuss it specifically until the mid-teen years.

• What is your immediate reaction when you think about sex? Do you feel happy, comfortable, anxious, sad, vulnerable, _____?

• How did you react emotionally to your first sexual encounter?

• Do you think men and women have different emotional connections to sex?

• How aware were you of the emotional side of sex before you became sexually active?

• What emotional changes do you think occur once someone becomes sexually active?

• Are there any emotions that you think are "negative" and should not be expressed?

• Do you think depression can be situational and triggered by events, or do you think it is a long-term condition triggered by genetics?

EXPLORING SEXUAL ORIENTATION

Identifying your thoughts about sexual orientation early on will allow you to plan how to talk about this delicate and sometimes controversial topic.

• Do you think of sexuality as fluid or static over the course of a lifetime?

- How do you think nature, including genetics and inherited traits, impacts sexuality?

- Do you think homosexuality is a choice?

- Have you ever felt attraction toward a member of your own sex, either in real life or in your fantasy life?

- What would your initial reaction be upon hearing that your child was gay?

EXPLORING COMMUNICATION

Thinking about your communication style is key in determining how you can best teach and connect with your child.

- Do you find it easy to actively listen to others? Do you think this is important?

- As a child, how did you receive criticism from your parents? How has this impacted your communication style as an adult?

- Do you feel a need to judge or weigh in on other people's decisions?

- What do you think is the best way to reprimand your child?

- What forms of discipline do you think are most effective?

- How do you think discipline should change as your child gets older?

- How involved do you think parents should be in their child's social—and eventually sexual—decision-making process?

- What do you think is the most effective way to communicate your family values about sex to your child?

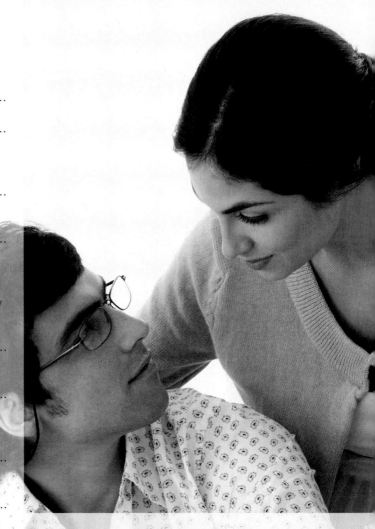

APPLYING YOUR ANSWERS Once you and your partner have discussed these answers you will feel more secure beginning a conversation about sexual thought and values with your child. If there are issues that you have very different viewpoints on—for example, homosexuality or how religion should impact sexual decisions—continue discussing until you are able to reach some compromise. These are big and sometimes controversial issues, and it is important that you are able to present one united viewpoint to your child, so as not to risk confusion.

Your child's mental development

Every child develops at a different rate mentally and emotionally, but there is a certain timeline of behavior that parents can expect. Note the four main stages of mental development and how these link to your child's sexual identity, then aim to establish an ongoing discussion about sexual health that corresponds with each stage.

Stages of cognitive development

As defined by the Swiss child psychologist Jean Piaget, there are four stages of cognitive development that a child moves through en route to adulthood. This means that your child is constantly being forced to adjust her view of the world in order to accommodate new pieces of information. Sometimes the information she receives ("The stove is hot") will only require a slight adjustment in her way of thinking ("Look out for the stove because it is hot"). However, there are times when new information requires a bigger adjustment in thinking and behavior, such as when she receives information about complicated concepts like anatomy or sex.

During each stage of her development, your child will process information differently, which means that the same facts might impact her in different ways depending on her age. Knowing this can help you tailor information to be truly age-appropriate and to match the processing level of each stage. The primary stages your child will go through are as follows:

Sensorimotor. From birth to age 2, your child's mental processes are derived from sensation and movement. During this stage, she learns that she is separate from her environment. She is object-oriented and repeats behaviors that are pleasurable to her.

This will most likely include touching and exploring her body, including her genitals. Children are born sensual beings. They thrive on being touched, stroked, kissed, and cuddled. The more your child connects with her body during this time and the more she is physically connected to and nurtured by her primary caretakers, the more secure and comfortable she will be in her body and self-worth.

Preoperational. From age 2 to age 6, your child is firmly focused on his own viewpoint, and believes that others see the world as he does. His thinking is also based on fantasy, or animism, in which inanimate objects are believed to have thoughts or feelings. He might believe that his favorite toy has human properties or emotions, for example. This is the stage where imaginary friendships are common.

"During each stage of development, your child will process information differently, so the same facts might impact her differently depending on age."

During this period you will find that your child is naturally and visibly curious about his body and his surroundings. It won't occur to him to feel self conscious about touching his body or genitals unless he receives negative feedback. Your child will also have firm beliefs about gender roles and will begin to identify the appropriate behaviors for his gender. The more permissive you can be during this time, the better, because this is the time when your child is really starting to make sense of his own body and gain a sense of agency and control over it. If he feels judged or anxious during this time, it can complicate his feelings of self-worth and value, as well as his body image.

Concrete operational. From age 6 to 12, your child is able to think logically. She is no longer ego-centric and is able to judge another person's viewpoint or feelings. She can solve problems and arrange and classify items. This is also the time when your child is starting to focus intently on peer relationships and fitting in. You may find, at least from ages 6–9, that she seems less focused on body self-exploration.

During this time, children also start to become very conscious of what is appropriate and inappropriate behavior. At around age 9 or 10, your child's social focus may start to include "boyfriends" or "girlfriends." Talk to your child about what these relationships mean and ask what boyfriends and girlfriends do together. Usually, these relationships are harmless and are simply about the title and trying adult ideas on for size. Relationships at this stage rarely include sexual contact or play, but if your child starts talking about this type of behavior to you or to her friends, check in with her about what this means and remind her about her private parts being private and that is not OK to touch someone else's private parts, or have them touch yours.

Your child is now able to logically understand the mechanics of sex, and by age 11 or 12, you can begin to explain how sex works in greater detail. As part of this conversation, it is a good

---

SEXPLANATION
WHAT DOES SEX MEAN?

Your child will think about sex in different ways as his mind develops. As he grows, general awareness of the mechanical process of sex will turn into a more personal identification with sexual thoughts and situations. He will begin to have highly individual questions, desires, and doubts associated with his own unique idea of sex.

SENSORIMOTOR, AGES 0–2: Your child has only abstract thoughts about sex.

- "Where do babies come from?"

PREOPERATIONAL, AGES 2–6: Your child will be fascinated by how twins are made, the logistics of an egg and sperm, and the idea that part "A" goes into part "B" in order for a baby to be made. He might think:

- "How do two babies grow inside a mommy's tummy?"
- "What happens when you have sex?"
- "How can the sperm find the egg?"

CONCRETE OPERATIONAL, AGES 6–12: Your child will consider how sex will impact her.

- "Will I grow up and have sex one day?"
- "Will I have babies?"
- "When will I get my period?"

FORMAL OPERATIONAL, AGES 12–15: Your child will begin to make decisions about sex, and will have more concerns and questions.

- "Am I the only one in my grade that is not having sex?"
- "Am I ready to have sex?"
- "I really want to have sex."
- "What if I am not good at sex?"
- "What if he or she laughs at my body?"

idea to also begin talking about sexually transmitted diseases and safer sex options, in addition to abstinence (see page 148). As you do this, you can reinforce your family values and clarify that you are simply providing important health information, not permission or encouragement to engage in any sort of sexual or intimate activity.

Formal Operational. Between the ages of 12 to 15 years old, your child develops the ability to think abstractly. He begins to fantasize about his future life, and also begins to change the way he thinks about social matters. Piaget termed this thinking "adolescent egocentrism." It involves a heightened sense of self-awareness, in which the child both imagines an audience is judging his behavior and feels an exaggerated sense of invincibility or uniqueness.

Adolescent egocentrism affects not only your child's general decision-making process, but also his sexual decisions. This is true for two reasons. First, he sees his behavior as being judged on a very large scale. Second, he feels an exaggerated sense of invincibility and uniqueness, which can lead to risky behavior. This could mean speeding down the highway at 80 mph, experimenting with drugs or alcohol, or engaging in unsafe sex. At this stage of development, the reality of STDs, pregnancy, and parenthood don't really hit home. Your child knows these dangers exist, and perhaps even know peers who have experienced them, but the threat isn't personal. Because of this, it is a good idea to frequently reinforce earlier lessons about safer sex and your family's values during this stage.

Receiving and processing sexual information

Even during the mid-teenage years, the young adult brain is not yet fully developed. The dorsal-lateral prefrontal cortex, which is the part of the brain believed to be responsible for judgment and consideration of risk, does not mature until your child is between the ages of 18-21. Its lack of development in adolescents may lead them to make risky or poor decisions.

An adolescent in this stage of development has plenty of mental cues that complicate her decision-making process, particularly as it relates to sex. She feels incredible pressure to fit in and impress her peers, she feels special and as though life's rules don't apply to her, and finally, this decision-making area of her brain isn't fully developed yet. Unfortunately, sex education doesn't tend to take these factors into account. Most schools focus on abstinence-only sex education, in which scare tactics are used to try and keep teens from having sex before they are ready. While the intentions are good, sex education that centers only on the dangers of sex isn't very useful for a teenager who sees those dangers as reserved for other people. A teenager who is still developing her decision-making skills and who feels invincible to risk will often find it very hard to listen to warnings about herpes and teenage pregnancy, particularly when hormones are running rampant. This is one of the primary reasons why it is a good idea to offer abstinence-based education rather than abstinence-only education.

"Sex education that centers only on the dangers of sex isn't very useful for a teenager who sees those dangers as reserved for other people."

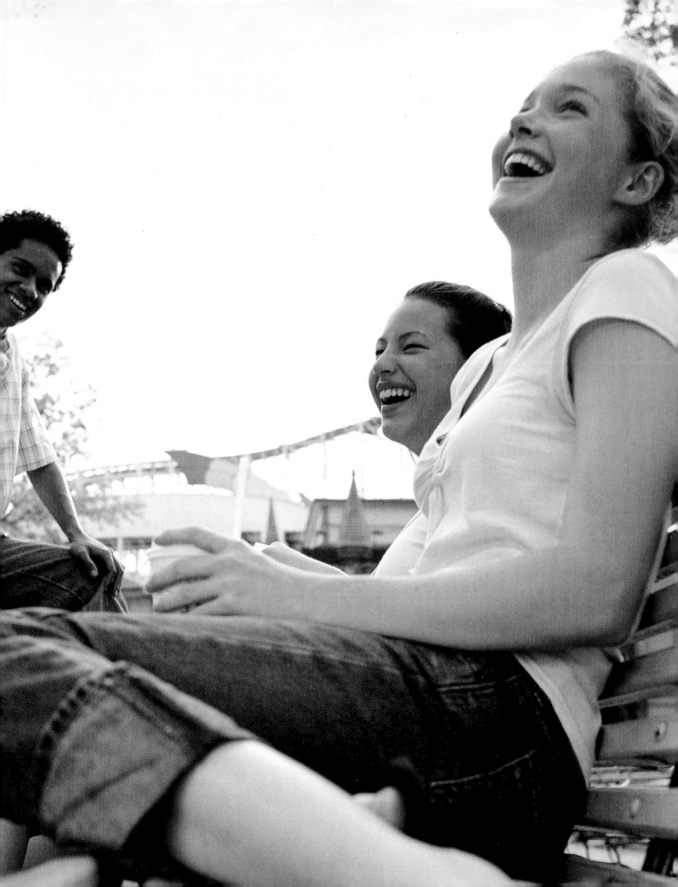

Discussing values

Your family values about sexuality will have an influential role in your child's sexual decisions, especially if you begin teaching these from a young age. Make this an open and ongoing dialogue, and your child will be more likely to think carefully about sex and to feel comfortable coming to you with questions and concerns throughout childhood and adolescence.

Sharing your values

Teachable moments that arise through the media or social situations can provide easy, natural opportunities to start a dialogue about your family's values, and ideally you will use these throughout your child's early years to start an ongoing conversation about sexual decision-making. However, as your child gets older it is also a good idea to set aside a specific time that you can devote to discussing your family values in greater depth. A planned conversation will help your child understand that this is a serious topic that is central to who you are as a family and to who she becomes as she grows up.

A good time to have this more formal conversation is when your child is around 11–12 years old. You can start the conversation by talking about how this is a special time in her life, and how excited you are that she is growing up. Then, let her know that because of this, there are some things you want to say to her.
For example, you might say: "I am so happy to see you becoming a beautiful young woman. This is such an exciting time—you are growing up, learning new things, and becoming an adult. Maybe you will fall in love with someone. You will also be faced with some adult decisions as you get older, and maybe you even have some friends who are having sex already. However, as you know, in our house, we believe in waiting to

have sex [until you are older, until you are married, etc]. The decision to wait isn't always easy, but I know that it is something that you will not regret doing."

It is also a good idea to talk to your child about responsibility as a sexual value. This will help her to associate smart sexual decisions—not sex itself—with maturity and adulthood, which are important ideals for adolescents. Explain that when you respect your body and are responsible about caring for yourself, you do not engage in unsafe sex, including sex that you are not emotionally prepared to handle. Let your child know that being responsible means more than just using a condom. It means being responsible for your own heart and your emotions, and the heart and emotions of your partner. If your child can understand that rushing into sex or having sex before she is ready is an irresponsible decision physically and mentally, she will be more likely to make careful and informed decisions about sex.

Expressing your values about waiting

As you share your family values, encourage your child to talk about his own feelings. If he shares that friends in his class are having sex already, or that he feels pressure to have sex, it is important to stress why waiting to have sex is part of your family's values. The temptation as parents is to stick to very simple reasons for postponing sex, such as "You aren't ready" or "Because it is the right thing to do." However, it is much more influential to be able to explain why waiting is important, not just why not waiting is wrong. Think about the primary lesson that you want your child to walk away with, such as that sex should be a well-thought out decision or that virginity is a valuable gift.

To express this, try saying something such as: "You probably have a lot of sexual feelings and desires, and that is all normal. However, I hope you know that your body and your sexuality are two of your most amazing and special gifts. This is why we value them so highly and are so careful about how we use these gifts."

Reflecting on sex

To make these values more personalized, it is a good idea to encourage your child to think about his own sexual values. The more your child thinks about values in a personal context, the more likely he will be to abide by standards that protect his body and his sexuality. He may also be more likely to make the connection between the physical pleasure of sex and the emotional responsibility that comes with it. You might want to consider giving your child a journal for this purpose, perhaps with a lock, so he feels safe writing down very private thoughts.

You can say something like: "I know we talk about sex a lot and we have a very open relationship, but as you get older, you will likely have some private thoughts about sex that you want to keep to yourself. I respect that and I am going to give you the privacy to think about these things for yourself. In the end, I can only help guide you in the right direction, and I can't make all of your choices for you. That is why it is important for you to spend time on your own, thinking or perhaps journaling about what you want in a relationship, and about your own sexual values. You might come across some questions as you are thinking, and you can come to me and talk about these whenever you want."

TEACHABLE MOMENT:
TALKING ABOUT SEX AND RELIGIOUS VALUES

If you are attending a synagogue, church, or mosque and there is a lesson on sexuality and morality, it is a good idea to follow up with your child after the service. Your child will probably have questions about some of the topics that were covered, particularly as it relates to her life now and in the future. If you aren't sure how to answer difficult questions (such as "If I have sex before marriage, am I going to hell?" or "I heard that Catholics can't use birth control. Does this mean I can't ever take the pill or use a condom?"), say that you will get back to her about this important question, then set aside time to meet with your religious leader to discuss ways of dealing with these doubts or concerns.

CONVERSATION STARTER 1: "That was an interesting service today, wasn't it. Do you have any questions about sex and morality? Did the rabbi address any issues that you have already been thinking about?"

CONVERSATION STARTER 2: "What did you think about the lesson we just heard? Have you and your friends ever talked about sex in the context of our religion? Do you think the guidelines the pastor mentioned make sense for people today, or do they seem dated and difficult to follow?"

Guiding decisions

In order for sexual values to take root, your child needs to be able to personalize these values. An important part of raising a sexually healthy child is helping her to form and embrace her own sexual identity. You can do this by helping your child process sexual information and values, and helping her reflect on what she wants out of a relationship, both in the present and the future.

Encouraging smart sexual decisions

When it comes to sex, helping foster positive decisions often begins by appealing to your child's sense of morality, though perhaps not in the way that you might expect. Remember that adolescents are able to think on an abstract level, so your child can process concepts such as love, as well as concepts such as purity or monogamy. Thus, while your child's decisions might still be complicated by feelings of invincibility, it is also a stage in which your child can think of abstract ideas such as true love and waiting for that "special someone."

Rather than using scare tactics to encourage your child to make smart sexual decisions, try to encourage these decisions through an ongoing dialogue about sex. This is ideally started much earlier in adolescence, because the earlier you begin this discussion with your child, the more time your values will have to sink in and become part of his own thought process and value system. Make sure the conversation is based on mutual give-and-take, and that you welcome your child's ideas and questions. The more open you are to hearing his ideas, the safer he will feel talking with you, and the more honest he can be about his fears and hopes. He will also be more likely to listen to you. This allows you to be more involved as he continues to process sexual information and feelings.

Talking about consequences

You can also teach positive decision-making by helping your child think through the possible consequences of her actions. Once your child envisions the entire path of consequences, she will be more likely to see how poor decisions can detract from her happiness. It is often useful to share personal experiences as a starting point for these conversations, so that you do not sound as if you are lecturing your child. For example, you can help your child understand that first love doesn't usually last forever by sharing about your first relationships.

Try saying something such as: "When I was your age, I was very in love with my first boyfriend. We thought we would be together forever, but we broke up during our junior year. At the time I was heartbroken, but within a few months I was already dating someone new. That's the nice thing about being young, there are so many people to meet and date."

You can then ask your child how long she imagines the relationship will last, and how she would feel if they had sex and then broke up. Helping your child to journey all the way down this kind of path—which may not occur to her otherwise—can help her understand the "what ifs" of the relationship and can help prevent any sexual decisions based on the idea that her first boyfriend is someone she will be with forever.

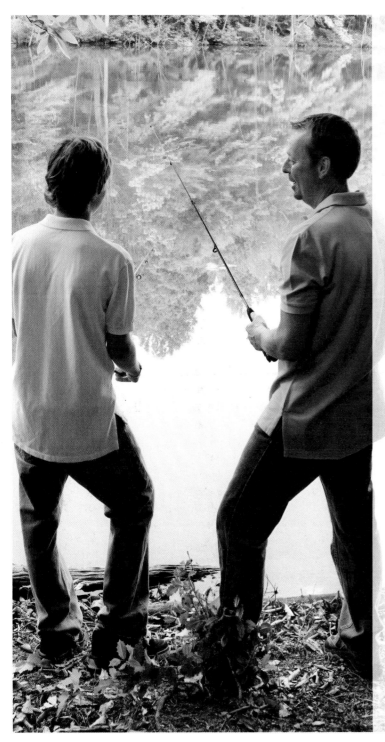

WHAT TO SAY . . .
IF YOU AND YOUR CHILD HAVE DIFFERENT VALUES ABOUT SEX

If you and your child have different values regarding sexuality and sexual activity, it can be difficult to find a middle ground. You can do so by agreeing to respect one another's opinions and come from a place of acceptance, rather than judgment. However, this doesn't mean that you should allow your child to make whatever decisions they want regarding sexual activity.

CONVERSATION STARTER: "I know you think you are ready to be sexually active, but I disagree. You can make your own decisions regarding your sex life when you are an adult (e.g. away at college, financially independent, etc.) but for now, I ask that you respect my feelings about this."

Give your child a chance to respond, then outline clearly what your response will be if he doesn't follow your family rules about sex.

FOLLOW-UP: If you break the house rules regarding sex, you will be punished, just as you would be punished for breaking the house rules regarding drinking or doing drugs.

Again, give your child a chance to respond. Close by reinforcing how much you want your child to have a happy sexual future.

FOLLOW-UP: "Unlike drinking or doing drugs, sexuality is a beautiful, experience that I want you to enjoy someday–but not until you are old enough to do so in a safe fashion."

Talking about sexual orientation

We are still discovering the natural, biological, and behavioral factors that affect sexual orientation. Because of this, it can be difficult to talk about this topic with your child—you likely won't feel as if you have all the answers. The important thing, however, is not being able to answer every question, but being open, direct, and respectful as you start this conversation.

The nature of homosexuality

There are many different viewpoints on the origin of sexual orientation, even within the medical and psychiatric field. In fact, it was not until 1986 that the American Psychiatric Association officially removed homosexuality from the *Diagnostic and Statistical Manual of Mental Disorders* (DSM). Up until that point, some homosexual behavior was still considered to be pathological and in need of medical treatment. However, we are now much better informed about homosexuality and sexual orientation, and know more about how genetics impact sexual identity and preferences.

Science shows that nature plays an important role in determining sexual attraction. Recent research may even point to a gene for homosexuality. A study led by a group of researchers at the University of Chicago isolated a gene that is involved in the sexual preference of fruit flies. If this gene is mutated, the fruit fly is bisexual and does not differentiate between male and female flies. Humans have a similar gene, although further research is needed to determine whether it has the same effect on sexual orientation. Still, this strongly suggests that sexual orientation is not a choice.

Other research suggests that sexuality might be related to birth order. Another study suggests that every time a mother gives birth to a son,

that son is progressively more likely to be gay. This is due to the levels of testosterone that develop in the baby's brain while in the womb. If a woman has already given birth to one or more sons, her body has lower testosterone levels to distribute to her next son's brain, which might affect his sexual orientation after birth. Indeed, studies have shown that each older brother increases his odds of developing a homosexual sexual orientation by 28-48 percent. Currently, there is no known correlation between a woman's birth order and her sexuality.

The nurture of homosexuality

Nurture may also play a large role in sexual orientation. Research shows that human sexuality is much more fluid than was originally thought. In fact, people can move across the sexual spectrum throughout their lives. For example, you might spend the first half of your life identifying as fully heterosexual, but then later discover strong bisexual leanings, perhaps as a result of meeting a member of the same sex you are very attracted to, or as a result of accepting buried sexual feelings and letting go of society's taboos. When people are honest and open to exploring their sexuality, it seems that only a small percentage of people identify as purely homosexual or purely heterosexual. This is true at every stage of life, and can be

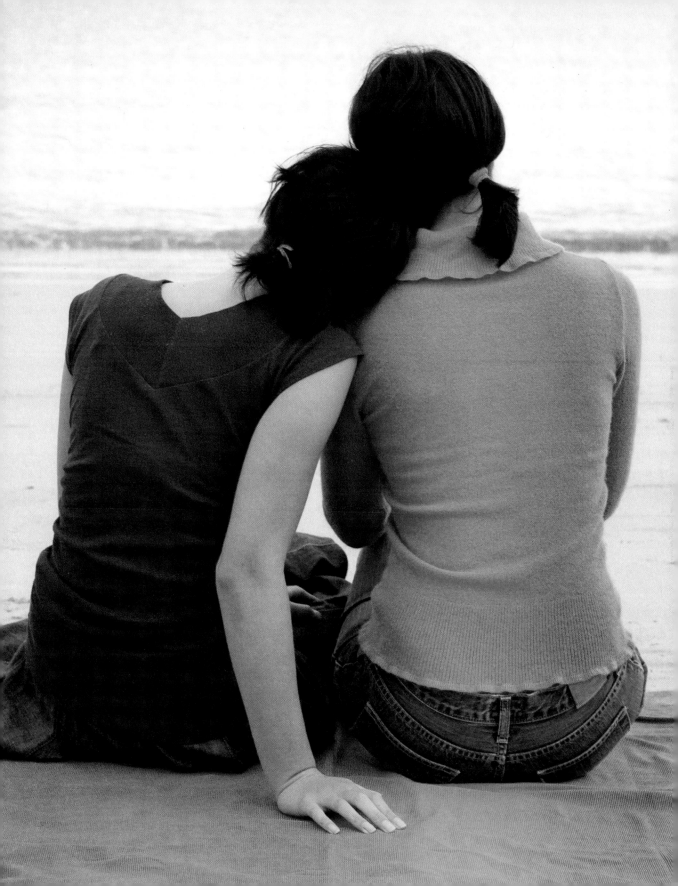

identified in same-sex childhood play, fantasies, and adult experimentation. Some studies suggest that women in particular have a fluid sexuality, in part because emotional connection can more easily translate to physical attraction.

Talking about alternate families

A good introduction to the idea of homosexuality is to talk with your child about how there are many different kinds of families. From a young age, let him know that some kids have two mommies, some two daddies, and some one of each. You might choose to do this when you see a homosexual couple on television or walking down the street. If you feel comfortable with this idea, let him know that it doesn't matter how a family is constructed as long as there is love and respect in the home; and point to examples you've seen on television or among friends, if possible. This can help your child grow into an accepting social citizen who won't judge his peers based on family systems or sexual orientation. Introducing the topic and helping him to feel comfortable discussing all types of sexuality will also make it more likely that he will come to you with any sexual orientation questions of his own.

You might say: "Just like people come in all shapes and sizes, families come in all shapes and sizes, too. Some kids have two mommies or two daddies. Some kids have one of each. And some kids have a mommy and a step-mommy, or a daddy and a step-daddy. It doesn't matter how they look, what matters is that they love each other."

Supporting a gay child

If your child identifies as homosexual, the best thing you can do is offer support and ensure that your home is a place that is loving and nonjudgmental. Gay and lesbian youth are more likely to commit suicide than other youths—in the United States, 30 percent of all completed youth suicides are related to the issue of sexual identity. Additionally, students who describe themselves as lesbian, gay, bisexual, or

---

TEACHABLE MOMENT
TALKING ABOUT HOMOSEXUALITY

A good way to start a conversation about homosexuality is to use a teachable moment, such as if you are watching television and come across an openly gay celebrity or a gay character. Say, "Did you know that [name of celebrity] is gay? Do you know what it means to be gay? Well, some people love men, and some people love women, and some people love both. For example, some girls have boyfriends, but some girls have girlfriends—or boys can have boyfriends or girlfriends. Love comes in all different forms. This can sometimes be controversial, but our family believes that It doesn't matter who you love, it just matters that you are happy."

CONVERSATION STARTER 1: "Have you and your friends ever talked about what it means to be gay? Are there any kids in your classes at school that seem to be interested in members of the same sex?"

CONVERSATION STARTER 2: "Do you remember my friend, Jason? He and his boyfriend love each other very much, and have a supportive and strong relationship, just like your father and I do. In fact, they probably have a more fulfilling family life then many more "traditional" couples who might not be so well-matched or loving toward each other."

transgendered are much more likely to miss school because of feeling unsafe, and are also more likely to engage in drug use and other risky or damaging behaviors.

Remember that regardless of your feelings on homosexuality, you can't control your child's sexual orientation. What you can do is help build her self-esteem. If you think your child may be gay, the most important thing is to let her know that you accept her no matter what. She might not readily admit that she is attracted to the same sex, but if you remain non-judgmental and keep the lines of communication open, it is more likely that she will open up to you at some point. To do this, it is a good idea to have a direct conversation with her about homosexuality, though this shouldn't take place until age 12 unless your child brings it up first.

You might say: "Remember when we talked about how there are all kinds of families and relationships? Sometimes a woman loves a woman, sometimes a man loves a man, and sometimes a man and a woman love each other. I just want you to know that whoever you are and whoever you love, I am always going to love you and be proud of you. If you have any questions or are confused about who you love or are sexually attracted to as you are growing up, you can always come to me."

Even if you have personal difficulties accepting your child's sexual orientation, it is crucial that you give her the support and compassion that she desperately requires during this time. Counseling can help your family learn to cope with this transition, as well as teach you communication techniques to keep your relationship with your child healthy. Also, many religious communities are starting to accept homosexuality and move beyond limited thinking, so if your family is religious, it might be a good idea to find a church or temple in your area that will accept your family and your child with love and compassion.

SEXPLANATION
WHAT IS THE RANGE OF HUMAN SEXUALITY?

The American biologist Alfred Kinsey suggested a way of examining sexual orientation that is now referred to as the "Kinsey scale" or the "sexual continuum." Kinsey's theory suggests that human sexuality is not as simple and straightforward as homosexual or heterosexual. Instead, our sexuality is fluid and open, and most of us have at least some incidental sexual interest in members of the same sex. In some of us, this might lay dormant and never come to light, and in others it might be present only as a minor fantasy in our sexual lives. Others who are higher up along the Kinsey scale (or who have a more open sexuality) might find that they are attracted to both genders to the point that they are bisexual. They might also find that their sexual preferences switch over time, so that where they were once attracted only to men, they are now attracted only to women. Those highest on the scale feel no attraction to members of the opposite sex.

RATING	DESCRIPTION
0	Exclusively heterosexual
1	Predominantly heterosexual; only incidentally homosexual
2	Predominantly heterosexual; but more than incidentally homosexual
3	Equally heterosexual and homosexual; also known as bisexual.
4	Predominantly homosexual; but more than incidentally heterosexual
5	Predominantly homosexual; only incidentally heterosexual
6	Exclusively homosexual

Puberty and emotional changes

Emotional changes and mood swings are an unavoidable part of puberty. Your child's increasing age and experience cause the inevitable process of growing up, and your relationship changes as a result. However, with patience and understanding you can establish a new, resilient bond with your older child that leads to an even more meaningful relationship.

Puberty and hormones

Emotionally speaking, the stages of puberty are difficult to define and calculate. However, it is common for adolescents to experience mild depression during this time. Hormonal fluctuations leave their bodies and minds feeling drained, which can cause changes in mood and leave teens feeling inexplicably angry or sad. They might lose their tempers more quickly and can be especially sensitive, becoming easily offended or hurt. While you don't want to cater to constant displays of emotion, it is a good idea to respond with extra understanding and patience during this time. Growing into a new, unfamiliar body while trying to figure out your place in the world around you is no easy task, and this is complicated by the stress and peer pressure all teens must deal with on some level. Ensuring that your child's home environment is supportive and loving can help minimize the emotional turmoil of this time, and can help prevent feelings of sadness or anger.

Dealing with mood swings

When you have a moody teen on your hands, try to realize that your thoughts are clearer than hers. The young adult brain is still developing, which means that her decision-making abilities aren't fully formed. Because of this, your child may deal with anger by slamming the door and screaming at you at the top of her lungs. An adult, of course, will look at this behavior and wonder: "What is she thinking?"

The answer is that she isn't—at least not to the degree that you are. In her mind, it seems like an appropriate way to deal with conflict, mainly because her judgment center isn't firing on all cylinders yet. This lack of judgment should not excuse bad behavior, but it does help you to know where your teenager is coming from: she isn't crazy—just highly emotional and running on hormones, not logic. Once you realize that your teen is responding to stress the best way she knows how, you can come at the situation with more patience and understanding.

"Ensuring that your child's home environment is supportive and loving can help minimize the emotional turmoil of this time."

Encouraging emotional release

The good news is that if you teach your teenager new ways to deal with her stress and emotion, you can prevent a lot of these blow-ups. One of the best ways to do this is to make your house a safe place to express emotion. This means that all emotions should be encouraged. Many of us think of emotions as either "positive" or "negative." We tend to shun emotions that we think of as negative, such as sadness, anxiety, or fear—all of which come with the territory for teens. However, the truth is that there is no such thing as a negative or a positive emotion. Every feeling is part of the human experience, and all are worth exploring and expressing.

It is when we don't explore these emotions that they can control us and cause bitterness or depression. Emotional outbursts tend to happen as a result of holding emotion in for too long, then releasing it at all once. If you encourage your teen to identify how she feels—whether it is sad, scared, afraid, or excited—and talk about it on a regular basis, you can minimize the likelihood of large-scale outbursts and also help her to learn how to identify and safely work through emotional turmoil.

Boys and emotions

Encouraging emotional expression is especially important when it comes to boys. Traditionally, young men grow up in an environment where the rule, spoken or unspoken, is that "boys don't cry" or "men don't get scared, they get even." Thus, when boys reach puberty and naturally begin to feel sad or scared, they don't feel safe expressing these emotions. Indeed, they might even feel guilty for having these feelings in the first place. This is why many young boys choose to lash out in anger or violence instead—they have learned that it is the only acceptable way for a man to express difficult emotions.

HOW TO ANSWER QUESTIONS ABOUT EMOTIONS DURING PUBERTY

Talk openly with your child about how she is feeling during puberty. Acknowledge that everyone experiences dramatic emotional responses sometimes, especially as they're growing up, and explain the science behind this as clearly as possible.

Q. Are hormones the reason I feel like crying for no reason?
A. Yes. Hormonal changes that happen with puberty can make you cry over small things that you didn't previously cry over. The good news is that your body will slowly adjust to the hormones and you will feel less emotional and more like yourself.

Q. Why do I need hormones if they make me feel sad?
A. You need hormones to help you grow into a healthy, strong adult. Even though hormones can make you feel bad sometimes, they are also a very important part of developing into a mature adult.

Q. Do hormones cause people to want to have sex?
A. In a way, yes. Hormones cause the body to develop physically, mentally, and sexually. However, just because your body is physically becoming more mature, that doesn't mean you are ready for sexual activity. In fact, hormones can cause you to have mood swings that might make it hard to make good choices, which is why you should wait until you are emotionally mature enough to make choices that aren't solely based on hormonal cues."

Help your child feel safe experiencing the whole range of human emotion by teaching him from a young age that crying is a healthy form of emotional release. Teach him also that boys sometimes feel scared, anxious, or depressed, and that all of this is normal. Let him know that the more he talks about these feelings, the better he will feel, and that it can be damaging to confine negative emotions inside of him. You can set an example in your own life by not being afraid to share emotion or be open, especially when with your family.

Getting through to your child

Simply stating that all emotions are accepted and healthy does not mean that your child will always tell you what he is feeling. Perhaps you read the previous section about making your home a safe place for emotion and thought, "But I do that already, and my teenager wants nothing to do with it. He won't talk to me about anything, let alone about his feelings." This separation is not unusual, and is in fact almost a required part of growing up. Your child is seeking his own identity and his hormones are driving him to want separation from authority.

A good way to help your child feel more comfortable about sharing with you is to allow him to choose when and how to express his emotions. Maybe he doesn't want to sit down and talk about how he is feeling, but he might feel comfortable doing so while you are both engaged in another activity. By staying open to the things he is interested in and not pressuring him to talk about his personal thoughts, you can show your teenager that you are invested in his life, but that you respect his need for privacy.

Try to find at least one thing you both enjoy doing together, such as playing video games, watching movies, or hiking, and keep it part of your regular traditions. In the midst of all the turmoil and change associated with growing up,

your child will like having one thing he can depend on to stay constant, such as your weekly tennis game or Sunday dinners. This will also provide a regular opportunity where your child may feel comfortable opening up to you without feeling pressure to talk.

If your teen still has a hard time opening up, try to ask him about how he is feeling, but don't push him. You can't force someone to be emotionally honest, you can only give guidance and allow space for sharing. Forcing your child to talk will only upset him and cause him to pull further away. If he is not receptive to your attempts at conversation, wait until another time and gently try to find out what's on his mind.

Increasing independence

Part of the reason that teenagers feel so frustrated during puberty is because they already feel like they have reached adulthood. While you know that your child is not yet ready to handle all of the responsibility that comes with being an adult, it is a good idea to recognize these feelings by giving her some freedom to make her own choices. You can limit this freedom by setting contingencies that her grades must remain high and her behavior must be in line, and outlining what form of discipline will occur if this does not happen. This type of limited responsibility will help her learn that her actions have specific consequences. By allowing your teen to make her own small-scale decisions, you will also help her to feel empowered, instead of frustrated and infantilized. This can go a long way toward improving her mood and behavior.

You might encourage your child to get a job so that she can afford her own transportation, or extend her curfew on weekend nights. You can also suggest that she start setting her own schedule, choosing when to do homework and when to take part in after-school activities.

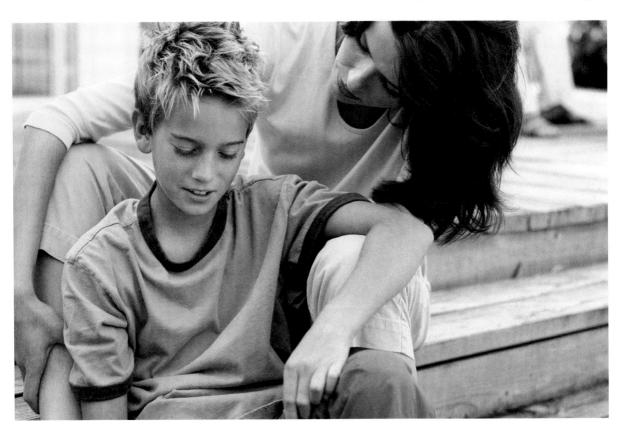

TEACHABLE MOMENT
TALKING ABOUT HOW TO EXPRESS EMOTION

When you notice your child is upset in some way, use the moment as a teaching tool to share how to deal with difficult emotions. First, explain how to use physical sensations to help identify emotions. For example, you can say that fear is generally accompanied by tightness in the chest, sadness with tingling in the eyes, and anger often leads to tense shoulders, back, or jaw. Find new ways to help your child release these emotions. For example, if he is angry, you might say: "Try releasing your feelings by hitting a pillow with a bat or screaming into a sink of water. This always makes me feel better. It is a good way to release difficult emotions without starting an argument."

CONVERSATION STARTER 1: "You seem angry this afternoon. Do you want to tell me about anything? Usually when I feel angry, my shoulders and back feel very tight because of all the tension that I keep there."

CONVERSATION STARTER 2:"It sounds like you had a really stressful day at school. One way to help release that stress is to find a physical form of release, such as going on a run or a long walk. Or you can even scream into a pillow or a closet, or somewhere else that is quiet and private. Just acknowledging that tension can help you feel much better."

LEARNING ABOUT CHANGING HORMONES

In addition to the physical developments of puberty, your child will need to cope with the emotional rollercoaster that hormones can cause for both boys and girls. This can be confusing for youngsters, who worry that they are the only ones dealing with these complex emotions. Help your child by reassuring her that she is not alone and that her changing feelings are just as normal as her changing body. It is a good idea to have this talk before puberty, around the ages of 9 or 10, but revisit the subject as you think necessary.

....

AFTER THIS LESSON YOUR CHILD WILL BE MORE LIKELY TO...

- Be able to identify what she is feeling and why
- Understand that it is normal to experience mood swings and intense emotions
- Accept that this is a temporary phase and that she won't always feel this way
- Feel more comfortable about expressing her emotions
- Investigate ways to cope with her emotions and feel better.

....

1 WHAT ARE HORMONES?

Does your child know that the word "hormone" means "to excite or stimulate"? That's what hormones do to your body. These chemical messengers circulate in your bloodstream and influence all your major bodily functions—from how tall you are to how much energy you have and how you respond to stress. You have more than 30 of these hormones busily orchestrating and regulating all of your bodily functions. Every time you get angry, become tired, laugh, cry, wake up, feel hungry, or fall asleep your body is responding to hormones. Many hormones are produced by your endocrine system, which includes your pituitary gland, pineal gland, thyroid, adrenal glands, and your testes or ovaries. There are also hormone-secreting cells in your digestive tract, kidneys, and pancreas. The hormones produced by the testes or ovaries are known as the sex hormones, and these are testosterone, progesterone, and estrogen. They are responsible for your child's development into sexual maturity. Growth hormone, produced in the pituitary gland, makes the body grow larger, sometimes very quickly. Arms and legs get longer and the internal organs increase in size, too. Hormones also affect the emotions. Even adults have to endure the effects of hormones, which can make a person feel happy or sad, spark aggression or anxiety, and affect the appetite or cause cravings for certain foods, especially sugar and other carbohydrates. During adolescence, your hormones are in overdrive, which means the effects are more exaggerated, and this can be difficult for adolescents to cope with.

2 HOW DO HORMONES AFFECT YOUR FEELINGS?

Does your child know how changing hormones are likely to make her feel? If she is currently going through puberty, she will probably be able to identify a range of difficult emotions. Explain that these are caused by the rapid and abrupt release of hormones into her body. Encourage your child to open up about her feelings. Is she feeling emotions more intensely? Perhaps she disliked something before and now she detests it, for example, or she used to feel sadness and now feels completely depressed on a regular basis. In addition to these stronger emotions, her moods are likely to swing wildly. Does she feel like she is brimming with happiness one minute, and bawling her eyes out the next? Does she feel extra-sensitive to criticism, to teasing—or to just about anything? Is she convinced that no one understands her, even the people closest to her? All of these responses can be triggered by hormones.

3 HOW LONG WILL IT LAST?

You can reassure your child that what she is experiencing is a temporary imbalance. Hormones normally settle down in time. Meanwhile it's important that she realizes that she is not alone. Let her know that even people who seem like they have it all together probably struggle with the same feelings from time to time. Try to help her see that although she may feel awful at a given time, the feelings will pass. If she does feel bad or worried all the time, however, it is not healthy for her to keep that to herself. Ask her to talk to you, and let her know that you will do your best to help.

4 CAN EMOTIONS BE CONTROLLED?

Talk to your child about strategies to help her cope with her emotions and mood swings. Suggest, perhaps, that she talk to trusted friends of her own age about how she is feeling. They might be feeling the same way, or know how to help her. At the very least they will be able to listen, empathize, and provide an outlet for her to let off steam. It is also a good idea to encourage her to find a creative outlet for her emotions. If she likes to draw, paint, write, play music, or sing, for example, these pursuits can be a good way to channel all that teenage angst. Even writing in a journal and giving expression to feelings can take the edge off them.

5 WHAT ELSE CAN HELP MINIMIZE OR PREVENT NEGATIVE EMOTIONS?

Eating healthily is a good way to help direct emotions, since mood swings can be made worse by too many processed or sugary foods. A balanced mix of all the food groups, such as fruits, vegetables, grains, and protein, will help give your child energy and prevent her from feeling tired and low. Keep a supply of fruit and healthy snacks at home so that your child is not as tempted to snack on unhealthy foods. Iron-rich foods, such as green leafy vegetables, lean meat, and beans, are also good for girls who are menstruating—a time when stressful emotions are often at their peak—since they lose iron in their blood each month. As you stress the connection between nutrition and hormones, make sure to reassure your child that her body is beautiful, and that she should eat well to stay strong and healthy, not to lose excessive amounts of weight.

HOW TO ANSWER QUESTIONS ABOUT CHANGING HORMONES

Deal sympathetically with questions, asking if there is anything the two of you can do together to make coping with hormones easier. Reassure your child that you love her. She may not show it, but children need to know they are loved more than ever during this very turbulent time. If your child won't talk to you, encourage her to talk to an older sibling, your spouse, a family friend, or perhaps even a religious leader or counselor.

Q. Why do I feel like no one understands me?
A. This is a time when you're likely to feel overly sensitive and sometimes see things out of proportion. It's part of growing up and forging your identity, but it won't last forever.

Q. Why can't I control emotions?
A. Remember that you are the one in charge and that you don't have to act on your feelings. This can help you feel more confident as you begin to get to know the exciting "new you."

Learning together

Encouraging open communication

Sometimes it seems like the last thing teenagers want from their parents is connection; instead, they want distance—and plenty of it! This is a natural part of growing up, but with the proper communication tools, you can create a strong and open relationship that lasts through the most difficult years of adolescence.

Communicating with your child

An important rule for communicating with your child is to talk with him, rather than at him. The moment you begin lecturing is the very moment your child will stop listening. Instead of nagging or yelling, frame your communication in a helpful and considerate manner. Always give your child a chance to respond, and when you are wrong, admit it and apologize. Communicate with your teen as you would with an equal, and treat him as someone whose opinion you value and whose feelings you respect. Stay calm even when you are upset about his behavior.

Try saying something such as "I've noticed that your grades have suffered over the past few months. Let's talk about why this has happened and what the consequences are going to be if they do not improve."

Listening to your child is equally important. One of the main complaints that teenagers have is that their parents don't listen to them. It isn't always easy to turn off the noise of the outside world and really listen—but once you start, you will be amazed at the difference it makes in your relationship with your teen.

If your child tells you that she feels as though you aren't listening, treat her opinion with respect. If possible, set aside time to talk immediately, and ask about the specific ways she feels unheard. During this conversation, listen closely, practice open body language, and ask questions that relate to specific concerns she raises. When she has finished sharing, it is a good idea to summarize the message back to her, so that you can make sure you are both on the same page and that you understand clearly why she is feeling upset.

>>> YOUR CHILD MIGHT BE SUFFERING FROM DEPRESSION IF . . .

Even the most involved parents find that their children sometimes will not open up and talk to them. A child who withdraws from the rest of the family might just be going through growing pains, but he might also be dealing with some very real emotional trauma. For this reason, it is important not to let signs of sadness go untreated or unnoticed. Your child might be suffering from depression if:

• He regularly appears anxious or angry
• His sleeping and eating habits have changed noticeably
• He has lost interest in his grades, or in hanging out with his friends

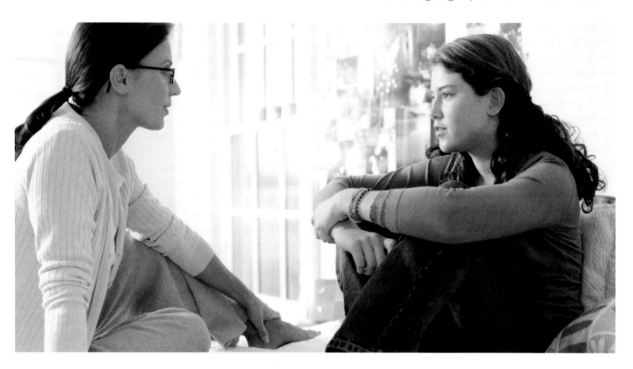

Giving negative feedback

Discipline and critique is a part of teaching your child what it means to be a responsible adult. The way in which you do this can make all the difference in the quality of your relationship and in your child's self-esteem. If you criticize or insult him, you will reinforce any negative feelings that he might be carrying inside. Thus, he may come away feeling as though he doesn't belong or always makes mistakes.

Instead, give your teenager negative feedback. Negative feedback means that instead of attacking the person who did something wrong, you explain what he did wrong and offer feedback on how to fix it. It means you are critiquing the action, not the person. Rather than insulting your child or yelling at him, try explaining what he did wrong and how he can fix it in the future. You can also outline for him what the consequences will be if he doesn't choose to do as he's been asked.

For example, you might say: "I asked you to take the trash out five times. When you don't listen to me, it makes me feel disrespected and it also makes me think that you don't appreciate me. I want you to take the trash out and contribute to this household. If you don't, I am not letting you go out tonight."

Avoiding judgment

It is very difficult to create an open, honest environment in your home while passing judgment on your teenager or on the world around you. Be careful not to send contradictory messages. If you tell your teenager that she can come and talk to you whenever she wants, but, for example, also regularly use condemning words like "whore" or "slut," your teenager will probably not feel safe coming to you with sexual fears or concerns. If you scorn other people's decisions, she will naturally worry that you will do the same to her.

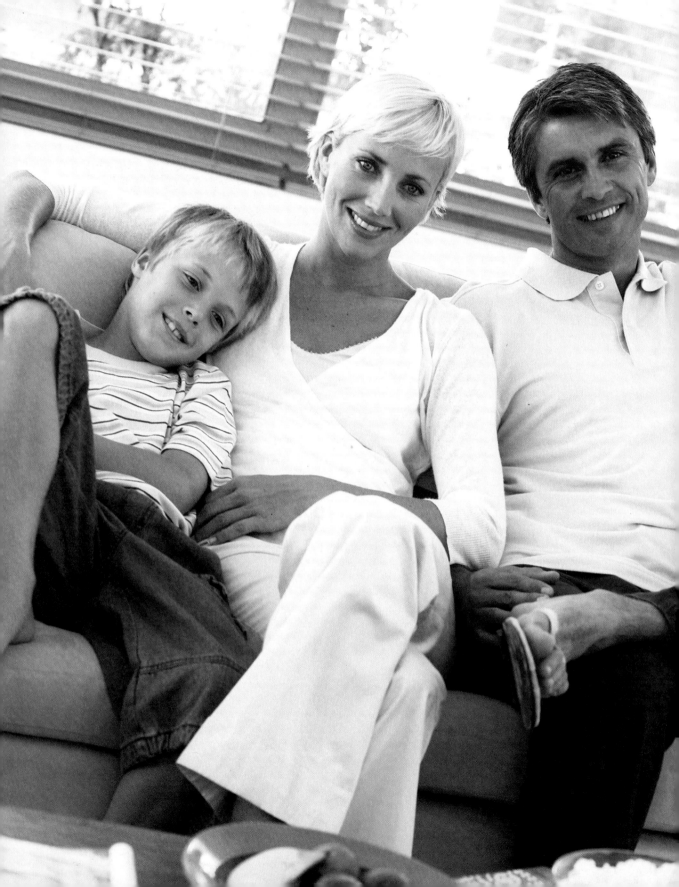

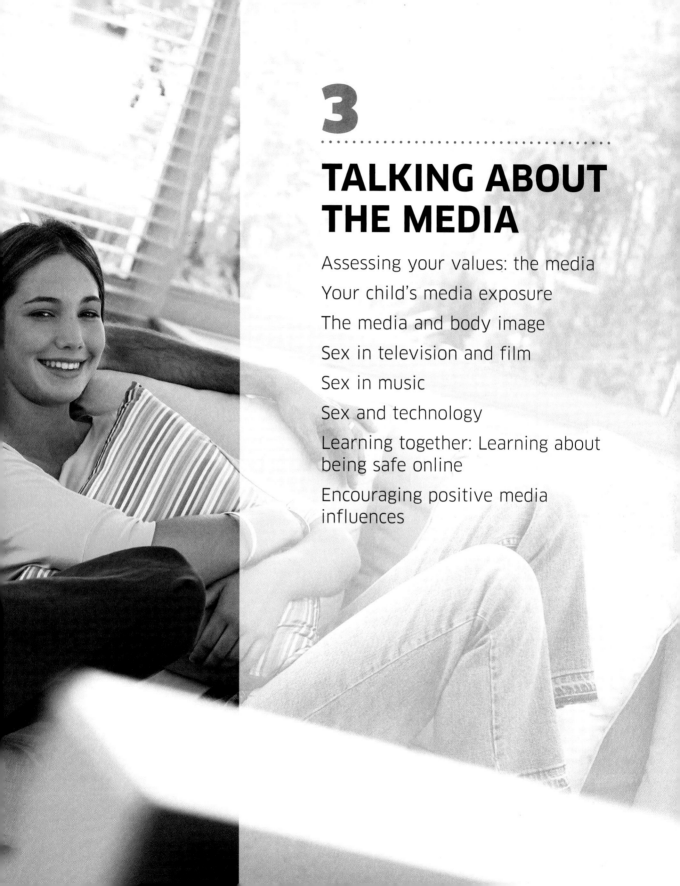

3

TALKING ABOUT THE MEDIA

ASSESSING YOUR VALUES: THE MEDIA

Media messaging is pervasive in our culture and the messages seem to be commanding our actions – buy this, wear this, eat this, drink this, listen to this, and of course, do this. As a parent, these messages have been shaping your identity since childhood. This gives you a lifetime of experience to draw upon when planning your child's media exposure. Think about the questions below privately, then talk with your partner about how to ensure that your child grows up in a safe and instructive media culture.

EXPLORING MEDIA AWARENESS

Staying informed about what's happening in the media world becomes important as your child grows and begins to identify more closely with what he is watching, reading, and hearing. Reflect on these questions to determine your level of awareness.

• In what ways do you think television and movies are valuable? How have they impacted you as both a child and an adult?

• How do you feel about TV programming today? What rules should be set about watching television inside and outside the home?

• How aware are you of current musical trends, and what do you think about popular music?

• Should your child be allowed to listen to music with sexually explicit lyrics? If so, at what age do you think this is appropriate?

• What do you think about networking sites such as Facebook or Twitter? Should there be any restrictions on your child's profile?

• In what ways do you think the Internet is valuable, and in what ways is it dangerous? How much time do you spend online?

• What rules should be set about Internet use?

EXPLORING MEDIA MONITORING

Monitoring your child's media influences can strengthen your relationship by keeping you better connected to your child's world. How strictly you supervise may depend on your child's interests and maturity level, and on the media monitoring you experienced as a child.

• How closely was your exposure to media monitored as a child?

• Do you monitor how much time your child spends in front of the TV or computer? How has this differed as she has grown older?

• At what age do you think your child should be able to make her own decisions about which shows to watch or which music to listen to?

• Do you think it's appropriate to monitor the books your child reads for adult content? What about magazines, including celebrity and fashion magazines?

• Do you think it's appropriate to monitor your child's cell phone usage, including picture and text messaging? Is this an invasion of privacy or a necessary evil in today's world?

• Do you think your child should be allowed to have a television or a computer in her room? If so, at what age is this appropriate?

EXPLORING MEDIA IMPACT

The media impacts all of us in ways we often don't think about. You can help your child keep a realistic perspective by identifying what media influences impact you positively and negatively, and discuss between yourselves in advance how to shape the impact that the media has on your child.

• Which type of media has the most impact on you (e.g. television, film, books, music)?

• Overall, do you think the media has a positive or a negative impact on your self-esteem and perspective of the world?

• What do you think about how the media (in particular, celebrity gossip and fashion magazines) portrays body image?

• How does this portrayal affect you? How do you think it may affect your child?

• How does the media affect your perception of sex and romantic relationships?

• How do you think it affects your child's perception of sex and romance, or your child's perception of the world in general?

• How do romantic scenes in movies impact your expectations for your own relationship? What impact did these have on you as a child?

• What impact does music have on you, and how does it influence your mood and the way you view others?

• Has increased access to the Internet, including social networking sites and chat rooms, impacted you as an adult?

• Do you think you can be overexposed to the media, and is this dangerous?

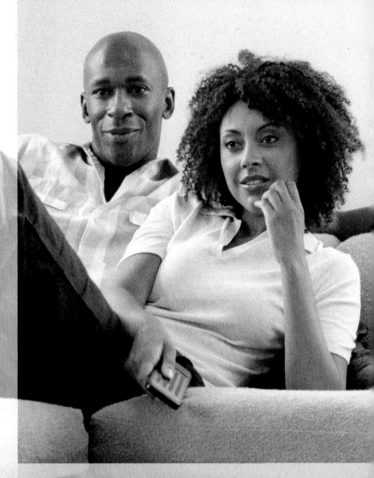

APPLYING YOUR ANSWERS Once you reflect on the far-reaching impact of the media, and the ways in which it influences you, you may find that your ideas about how to monitor your child's media exposure begin to change. In fact, you may also find that elements of your own media exposure are damaging your self-esteem or encouraging unrealistic relationship expectations. After determining which media influences are positive and informational, you will be well-equipped to begin educating your child on this influential part of social culture.

Your child's media exposure

There is no denying the power of the media. The trick as a parent is to separate the good influences from the bad, to ensure that the media contributes to your child's healthy self-image and to an equally healthy view of sex and relationships. Minimize media risks by monitoring your child's exposure, limiting and directing use, and seeking out positive programming.

The prevalence of the media

Many children today grow up with televisions in their bedrooms. They can watch a wide range of programming from their personal computers, fulfilling just about any search. They have cell phones and portable media devices and instant access to gossip and chat rooms and even pornography. They read magazines and blogs and the profiles of friends and strangers online. Media influences are truly everywhere.

This is valuable in many ways, but it is also scary for parents. With media this prevalent, it is hard to know exactly what programming your child is watching. Today's media includes sex, violence, coarse language, and adult situations as a matter of course. Finding age-appropriate content becomes a greater challenge every year.

The influence of the media

Research shows that adolescents who watch television with sexual content or listen to music with sexually explicit lyrics are more likely to engage in unsafe sex. These children are also more likely to become sexually active at a younger age than those who are not so exposed.

When young adolescents witness sexual content, they are often unable to put the situations in the context of their values. As a result, children are more likely to be swayed into engaging in sex before they are ready. While sexual content does not create sexual feelings, it does bring these feelings to the surface and can encourage exploration.

This doesn't mean that children who are allowed to watch whatever they want cannot grow into healthy, responsible adults, but it is a big risk to take. Too much media exposure can fast-forward your child's learning curve for topics that he may not yet be able to fully process. Limiting this exposure is an important responsibility of parenthood. If you discover that your child has watched, read, or listened to something with adult content, find time to talk to him about it and ask if he has any questions.

Creating a media plan

It is a good idea to sit down with your partner and talk about the restrictions you want to set for your child's media exposure. Having specific rules in place can help make boundaries fair and expected for your child. For example, you might discuss when your child will be allowed to have a social networking profile, or when she will get her own cell phone. Think also about the boundaries you want to set around shows with violence, sex, and other adult content. There is no right or wrong answer to these questions—each family has to find what works best for them and what suits their child's maturity level.

Limiting your child's media exposure

It is a good idea to start monitoring your child's media exposure from an early age. If limited television, movie, or computer rights are routine, your child will be less likely to view them as punishment. Begin by placing all televisions and computers in common areas, not in your child's bedroom. Late-night television watching or Internet surfing can disrupt sleep and potentially affect grades, and it will also make it easier for your child to be exposed to programming that is too adult. Having your television and computer in a centralized location like the living room where you can keep an eye on everything that comes onscreen is a simple way to monitor media exposure. You can supervise even more closely by inquiring with your cable company about which parental blocks are offered.

You can also limit your child's media exposure by only allowing a few hours of television each week, such as Saturday morning cartoons or Friday night movies. While it might seem standard for children to play video games and watch television all night, remember that you can decide to set much stricter limits than this for your child. Constant media exposure will not only affect your child's potential sexual decisions, it may also chip away at intelligence and creativity. Thus, it is a good idea to make TV and movies a treat, rather than a right.

Monitoring older children

Limiting a young child's media exposure is not very difficult, since you have a good deal of control over his daily activities. However, as your child gets older and begins spending time at friends' houses or watching television and playing on the computer alone, you lose some of your ability to monitor what he sees. Talk to your child about the new freedom he has received, and the responsibility that goes along with it. **For example, you might say:** "Your father and I are so proud of how hard you have been working in school. We want you to have more freedom and be able to watch TV on your own or at your friends' houses. But it's important that you still follow the house rules, even when there's no supervision. Remember that it's not okay to watch R-rated movies. If we can trust you to follow our rules, we can give you more freedom as you get older. If not, we might have to take some of your privileges away."

>>> YOUR CHILD IS BEING INFLUENCED BY THE MEDIA WHEN . . .

How early your child begins to internalize content from television, movies, or music depends on how much exposure your child has to the media. Precocious questions or comments are usually the first sign of this—and while these might be good for a laugh later with your partner, remember they also signal that your child might be starting to have questions or concerns about sex that should be discussed. Specific signs include:

• Using four-letter words that mimic curses heard on television—often the first sign that the media is a real influence
• Spending considerable time watching television or movies with an older sibling who watches more adult programming
• Questions about adult ideas, such as: "What does sexy mean?" or "What did that lady on TV mean when she said foreplay?"

The media and body image

It is no secret that the media worships slimness and beauty. As a parent, you have probably experienced your own insecurities because of this. To protect your child's self-image and view of sexuality, the important thing is to seek out media sources with realistic figures, give your child regular positive feedback, and set a good example with the things you personally watch and read.

The media, body image, and self-esteem

The media can boost or damage self-esteem, particularly for children who are engrossed in discovering their identity. For adolescents, defining identity is as much a process of social discovery as it is a process of self-discovery—in order to know who they are, children first want to know who everyone else is. A large part of this discovery process requires that children compare their own identities with those that they see reflected on television and in the movies, which can sometimes lead to feelings of low self-worth and poor body image. In turn, a poor body image can lead to a decreased self-confidence and an increased chance of engaging in unsafe sexual activity.

One notable study found that young women reported having a significantly lower body image after viewing very thin media images than after observing "average" or plus size models. This effect was felt most intently by women under 19 years of age, which is the stage when young girls are growing into their adult bodies. Around this age, girls naturally compare their bodies to the bodies of models in magazines and on television—and often find themselves inferior.

It isn't just girls who are struggling with body image. Both boys and girls who identified with TV stars and boys who identified with athletes were found to have higher levels of dissatisfaction with their bodies. In fact, another study has found that media messaging can cause boys to try and change their physical appearance. Australia's Deakin University interviewed boys from ages 12 to 15 and found that media messages affected the boys' desire to alter their body size through exercise and physical training.

Poor body image contributes to low self-esteem and emotional distress—and this can start from an early age. Part of the reason that body image is so crucial to a healthy self-esteem is because the media often equates goodness with thinness and beauty. A recent study found that attractiveness and thinness are associated with goodness in over 100 female characters

"The media can either boost or damage self-esteem, particularly for children who are engrossed in discovering their identity."

appearing in 23 Walt Disney animated films. For example, in Cinderella, the ugly stepmother and rotund stepsisters have evil characters, while the good and noble heroine is beautiful and thin. This theme recurs often in these and other children's stories, causing young viewers to learn from an early age that to be beautiful is to be good, while to be ugly is to be bad.

Counteracting negative messages

The results of all of these studies have one thing in common—they show how greatly the media can affect the way your child feels about herself. Combating these many images isn't easy, especially when negative messaging begins at an early age.

This doesn't mean that you have to prevent your child from watching animated classics, or from reading magazines and following the media coverage of athletes and celebrities. Giving your child plenty of positive commentary is one of the best ways to keep self-esteem high and prevent her from seeking attention in other ways, such as unsafe relationships or sexual activity.Compliments alone can go a long way in diminishing the destructive power of the media. The Deakin University study, for example, found that complimentary feedback had a positive impact on helping to build up boys' self-esteem. However, it didn't completely counteract negative media influences.

Finding positive media influences is also a good way to inspire healthy self-esteem in your child. Try to focus on television shows that illustrate values you want your child to emulate, and also seek out programs that don't put emphasis solely on how people look. Look for characters that are multi-dimensional and can help teach your child that character is much more important than beauty, as well as for characters that value sincere love and close relationships, rather than casual sex.

TEACHABLE MOMENTS
TALKING ABOUT MEDIA IMAGES

As your child grows older, she will become more and more aware of images she sees in magazines and on television—many of which are unhealthily thin. Take advantage of these moments to reassure your child that these are not realistic images, and that Hollywood often uses airbrushing, creative lighting, and hair and makeup artists to create false perfection. Simply making a point to state these truths out loud can play a huge part in counteracting unrealistic messages about the body. For example, you might say: "I noticed you were looking at fashion magazines with your friends today. Sometimes when I look at magazines like that, it makes me feel bad about my own body. But, then I remember that the reason those models look so perfect is because they are airbrushed and digitally manipulated to look that way. I think true beauty is someone who is healthy and confident and smart—just like you!"

• **ALSO MAKE IT A POINT TO** praise real and healthy body types, such as strong female athletes. Teach your child that bodies come in all different shapes and sizes, and that each one is special, attractive, and most importantly, unique. Celebrate real, natural beauty and make confidence the ultimate goal, both in your own life and in your child's life.

CONVERSATION STARTER 1: "Isn't it fun to watch the women's tennis finals? The athletes are so strong and well-toned. What a difference compared to the women you sometimes see on TV—I think these athletic women are much more beautiful and real."

CONVERSATION STARTER 2: "The people in [insert name of show] are really good-looking. But I bet even they have days when they feel ugly, especially when they don't have make-up artists and stylists to help them."

Sex in television and film

There are ways to guard against TV and film becoming a primary influence in your child's life. Protect your child against mature content by monitoring when and where she watches TV, blocking inappropriate shows, and talking about how the behavior she sees onscreen can be unhealthy and sometimes even dangerous.

Blocking content

The first step is to agree with your partner about what television shows and movies are age-appropriate. If you need a guideline, consult your V-Chip ratings. The V-chip is an electronic component already contained within many television sets. It allows programs to be filtered according to established ratings that gauge the explicitness of content, by allowing you to set a password that restricts access to certain programming. This device was created just for the purpose of preventing children from seeing sex, violence, and other unsuitable content.

Take advantage of the V-chip as a directional tool, but don't become a slave to its ratings. If your child wants to watch a show that has been blocked, try watching it on your own first before agreeing to let him watch it. Ultimately, these ratings are just general guidelines. Every child develops and matures at a different rate, and you are the best judge when it comes to what material your child can process.

When you do use your V-chip, you'll may notice additional letters next to the basic rating, which indicate that a show contains higher levels of violence, sex, or adult language. These letters have the following meanings: V—violence, S—sexual situations, L—coarse, crude, or indecent language, D—suggestive dialogue (usually means talk about sex), FV—Fantasy violence. In addition, the formal V-chip ratings are:

TV Y—All Children Content is appropriate for all children, and all themes and elements are designed specifically for a young audience, including children aged 2-6.
What you need to know: Not all TV-Y shows are violence-free. Some shows with cartoon violence are rated TV-Y, such as the "Road Runner" cartoons. There is no content rating to let you know if a TV-Y show contains violence.

TV Y7—Older Children These programs are designed for children ages 7 and older, and may require the developmental skills needed to distinguish between make-believe and reality. Themes and elements may include mild fantasy or comedic violence, so may frighten or be unsuitable for younger children.
What you need to know: TV-Y7 shows that contain high levels of fantasy violence are supposed to be labeled with the "FV" rating. But even some TV-Y7 shows without the FV label may contain violence that could be of concern to parents, although it is usually much milder than in shows with the FV label.

TV Y7 FV—Older Children-Fantasy Violence Programs that contain more intense or combative fantasy violence are given this label.
What you need to know: A TV-Y7-FV rating indicates a program that may contain some or all of the following characteristics: violence as a prevalent feature of the program; fighting

presented in an exciting or thrilling-way; villains and superheros valued for their combat abilities; violent acts glorified; and violence depicted as an acceptable or effective solution to a problem. Fantasy violence may be part of an animated cartoon, a live-action show, or a program that combines both animation and live-action.

TV G—General Audience Generally appropriate for all ages. Programs with this rating are not designed specifically for children, but they contain little or no violence, no strong language, and little or no sexual dialogue or situations.
What you need to know: Most TV-G shows don't contain any sex, violence, or adult language at all. However, there are no content ratings used on TV-G programming to let you know if shows do contain such content.

TV PG—Parental Guidance Suggested This programming may be inappropriate for young children due to the following: moderate violence (V), some sexual situations (S), infrequent coarse language (L), or some suggestive dialogue (D).

What you need to know: Many TV-PG shows do contain moderate levels of sexual dialogue or violence, and not all of them are labeled with the content ratings. TV-PG shows with higher levels of sex, violence, or adult language are usually identified with content labels.

TV14—Parents Strongly Cautioned This programming contains some content that is unsuitable for children under the age of 14, and should be monitored for younger children. It may contain one or more of the following: intense violence (V), intense sexual situations (S), strong coarse language (L), or intensely suggestive dialogue (D).
What you need to know: Most TV-14 shows contain sex, violence, or adult language. Not all of those shows are labeled with the content descriptors. TV-14 programs with the highest levels of sex, violence, or adult language are usually labeled with the content ratings. A TV-14 rating without content labels may also indicate a program with a mature theme. It is a good idea to monitor these programs as much as possible.

TEACHABLE MOMENT
TALKING ABOUT TEEN PREGNANCY IN THE MEDIA

Teen celebrity pregnancies seem to have become a virtual epidemic. Many parents fear that this will make teenage pregnancy look cool or trendy to their children, but you can actually use these situations as a parenting tool to encourage your child to talk about teenage pregnancy. For example, try saying "I hear that [insert celeb's name] is pregnant. She is only 16 years old. I think that she and her boyfriend have chosen a very hard path. What do you think about teens having babies when they are so young?" Listen to your child, and don't judge his reaction. The point is to create a safe place where your child can express fears or concerns without feeling attacked.

CONVERSATION STARTER 1: "Do you know anyone in your grade who has gotten pregnant or had a baby, like the girl we saw on TV? Do you ever think about what would happen if you got someone pregnant [became pregnant]?"

CONVERSATION STARTER 2: "It seems like more and more teenage couples are choosing to raise their child together. What do you think about that? Does it seem scary to be a parent at your age? Do you know any children that have made a similar choice?"

TV MA—Mature Audience Only This program is specifically designed to be viewed by adults, and may be unsuitable for children under the age of 17. This program may contain the following: graphic violence (V), explicit sexual activity (S), or crude or indecent language (L). **What you need to know:** Very few shows are labeled MA.

Monitoring content

As your child gets older, it will become less important to block content entirely and more important to monitor content. One of the best ways to do this is to sit down with your child and watch some of her favorite television programs. You might not be naturally interested in a young adult program about the trials and travails of high school, but by watching these shows you can help ensure that they are age-appropriate, and also gain valuable insight into your child's mind. Not only will you learn what types of things your child is currently interested in (fantasy, romance, adventure, comedy), you will also see more clearly the themes, fears, and emotions your child might be experiencing in her own life. Sitting next to her as she watches and responds to the show will help you gauge how she is feeling—does she seem intrigued by the romantic storyline, for instance? Or does she still believe that boys have cooties? Does she notice or respond to any innuendo about sex? All of these are important lessons that may be easiest to learn through media exposure. After the program is over, you can use it as a conversation starter.
For example, you might say "I noticed that Jessica on [insert television show] had a boyfriend. Do you know anyone in your grade that has a boyfriend?" Or, "In that show we watched together last night, Kelli seemed nervous about getting her period for the first time. Is this something you worry about?"

As much as possible, it is also important to monitor what your child watches when she is out of your home. If she is going to a slumber party for instance, remind her of your rules before the party. Talk together about how you are trusting her to have a night out of the house, and how if she breaks that trust by watching shows she isn't allowed to, it will prevent her from going to slumber parties in the future.
You can also stay involved by talking with the parent in charge about the types of shows your child is allowed to watch. You might say, "My daughter is so excited to come to your home for the slumber party. I hear the girls might watch some movies. In our house, we don't watch anything rated higher than PG. We just want to be sure she doesn't watch anything she isn't allowed to, and of course, we would be happy to have her bring over some DVDs that she is allowed to watch."

Discussing rules

As your child gets older, you will have to start reevaluating your rules around what he watches. Make your boundaries clear as early as possible and set benchmarks for his future freedoms. This will help him understand the reasons that these rules are in place, as well as teach what content is off-limits.
For example, you might say: "We don't want you watching any movies with a PG-13 rating until you are 14 years old. This is because these shows often contain adult language and situations. If you show maturity and that you can handle watching these movies without any behavioral issues, then we will keep giving you more freedom. By the same token, if you pick up bad habits from watching shows with more adult content—such as breaking your curfew or having girls over when you are home alone—then we will start to limit your television and movie watching again."

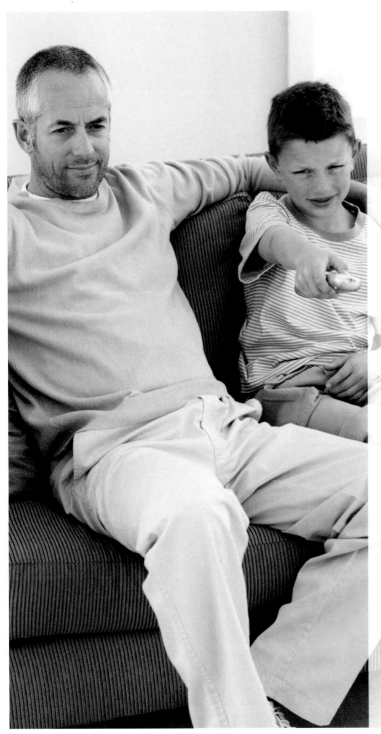

WHAT TO SAY . . .
TO SHAPE MEDIA MESSAGING

No matter how influential television messages are, your influence as a parent can be stronger if you maintain a regular dialogue about what your child is watching. An ongoing conversation will allow you to put your child's media influences into context and frame what she sees around your own family values.

CONVERSATION STARTER: "I know you like to watch [name of television program], but I think we should talk about some of the things the main character has been doing lately. In the latest episode, she thought about having sex with her boyfriend for the first time."

Give your child a chance to respond, then guide the conversation to become more personal.

FOLLOW-UP: "I know this is something that you are probably thinking about as well, and it's a normal and healthy part of growing up. But the decision to have sex is a big one, and I don't want you to make this big decision based on the TV shows you watch."

Emphasize the difference between what she sees on television and what happens in real life, then ask your child direct questions so she can become involved in the conversation.

FOLLOW-UP: As you know, those people are just actors, but your decision to have sex will have a lasting impact on you. When do you think is the right time to have sex? Do you and your friends talk about this?"

Sex in music

There is no discounting the pull of music, particularly over a young person who is searching for answers and looking to discover her own identity. As parents, it is a good idea to give your child enough distance to establish her own interests and tastes. At the same time, stay attuned to the messages of the lyrics your child listens to, and also to if and how they impact her behavior and self-image.

Lyrics and sexual messaging

What exactly is the music of this generation saying about sex—and does it really contribute to the sexual decisions of our youth? Recent research suggests that it might. A study led by RAND at the University of Pennsylvania, part of an international research and development group, examined the link between the sexual activity of teenagers and the level of sexually explicit lyrics they listened to. In this study, sexually explicit lyrics were defined as lyrics that discussed sexual acts in detail. Specifically, the lyrics in question depicted men as bold, aggressive, and dominating and women as submissive, and obedient, roles that young listeners might later adopt as their own in relationships and in sexual situations.

The study found that teenagers who listen to music with sexually explicit lyrics are more likely to initiate intercourse, as well as more likely to progress to more advanced levels of non-coital sexual activity. In plain English, teens that regularly listen to explicit sexual lyrics are more likely to have sex, and are more likely to progress to other sexual acts, than teenagers who do not listen to such lyrics.

Of course, some might argue that teens that engage in sex at an earlier age are also more likely to enjoy music with sexually explicit lyrics. This could very well be true. However,

regardless of the relationship between cause and effect, one thing is for sure—teenagers who listen to music with sexually graphic lyrics are having sexual messages and even sexual imagery pounded into their brains. Whether they choose to act on these messages or not is up to them, of course, but logic suggests that the more a teenager listens to these lyrics, the more difficult it is to avoid temptation.

Monitoring music

One way to help limit the effect of destructive lyrics is to forbid this type of music in the home. It's particularly important to outlaw lyrics that depict women as passive, submissive sex objects built purely for a man's enjoyment. These messages can be dangerous for boys and girls—both might begin to internalize and possibly act on the dominant male/submissive female sexual stereotype, even if they are surrounded by a number of other positive messages.

Instead of simply setting rules, explain to your child why you are forbidding him from listening to certain songs or types of lyrics. **For example, you might say:** "These lyrics are not just inappropriate for someone your age—they are inappropriate for any age. Lyrics like these are hostile towards women [use an example of lyrics if necessary] and they glorify casual sex and alcohol abuse. I understand that you have your own taste in music, and I want you to explore that, but you need to find music with messages that we can support and that don't go against our family values."

Ultimately, restricting your child's freedom won't make him become the kind, just, and ethical person you want him to be. However, if you communicate to your child a sense of purpose and reasoning behind the rules you create and empower him to make smart decisions, your child will be more likely to choose not to listen to offensive or explicit music. Children have a very strong sense of right and wrong, and they can be passionate advocates against injustice. Explaining why certain lyrics are damaging will help protect against unsafe influences, and also encourage your child to understand social justice and responsibility from an early age.

Positive musical influences

While you want to prohibit sexually explicit and toxic music from your home, this doesn't mean that your teenager can't enjoy any popular music. In fact, the RAND study found that song lyrics that made more veiled references to sex did not have the same effect on a teenager's sexual decisions. Lyrics that portrayed sex as romantic or as part of being in love were not correlated with early or casual sexual behavior. This helps illustrate an important point: it's okay to talk or think about sex, as long as a central part of the message is that sex is meant to be respectful, mutually enjoyable, and for monogamous adults. In fact, sending these types of messages might even encourage your child to reflect on what it looks like to be in a healthy, supportive romantic relationship.

WHAT TO SAY . . .
IF YOU ARE DISTURBED BY YOUR CHILD'S MUSIC

Music preferences are often a matter of personal taste, and you and your child will certainly not enjoy all the same artists. However, if your child is listening to music that you think is not suitable for his age, perhaps because of sexually explicit or violent lyrics, ask him about it.

CONVERSATION STARTER: "You know, I listened to some of the lyrics on the [insert band name] CD. I am worried because some of the content was a little too explicit and violent for my taste."

If your child is unresponsive, be direct.

FOLLOW-UP: "Tell me why you like this group so much? What do these lyrics mean in your opinion? Do you agree with the things they have to say?

Sex and technology

Technology is a useful tool, but it can also be the gateway to information that your child is not yet ready to know. Each year, there are more opportunities for children to interact with sexually explicit material through the Internet, online social networks, and other IT advancements. Because of this, it is important to stay informed of the technology that impacts and influences your child.

Monitoring Internet activity

You can help your child make smart decisions when it comes to Internet use and other technology privileges by monitoring conduct from a young age. Don't be afraid to set rules: remind your child that privacy is a privilege, not a right, and that when it comes to the Internet there is no such thing as true privacy.

Stress appropriate Internet use by explaining that some material is for adults only. Direct your child to specific child-friendly sites, and place the computer in a visible area where you can be present to monitor usage. You can also set rules, such as: "You can use the Internet for an hour a day" or " No messaging with strangers."

In addition, it is a good idea to monitor how much time your child spends online and on the phone. Make a "no cell phones at dinner" rule or a "no email during family time" rule—and don't forget to stick by it as well. Setting aside non-technology time will allow you to stay connected as a family, which in itself is one of the best ways to protect against negative influences.

Guarding against risk

It is important to teach your child about the possible dangers of the Internet from an early age. This will ensure your child is aware of what type of information is inappropriate to share and to receive, and will also help teach what to look for in terms of sexual predators. Your child can more easily come to you if questionable contact is made if you have started the initial conversation by identifying actions, language, and online requests that are inappropriate.

Remind your child that other Internet users might not always be who they seem. They might claim to be fellow classmates or kids of the same age, but in reality, they might be much older adults, or even sexual predators. Teach your child that he should never give out personal information to strangers online, including school information, locations of social events, home address or phone number, or any passwords. It is also important to encourage your child not to chat, message, email, or have any virtual contact with someone online that he has never met in person.

Social networking sites

Social networking sites are online communities where members build profiles and share personal pictures, information, and details about their daily lives. For adolescents, these sites offer an authority-free world in which to communicate their own unique identity and connect with peers. Think of these social networking sites as a virtual mall—a mall with no parents and no supervision.

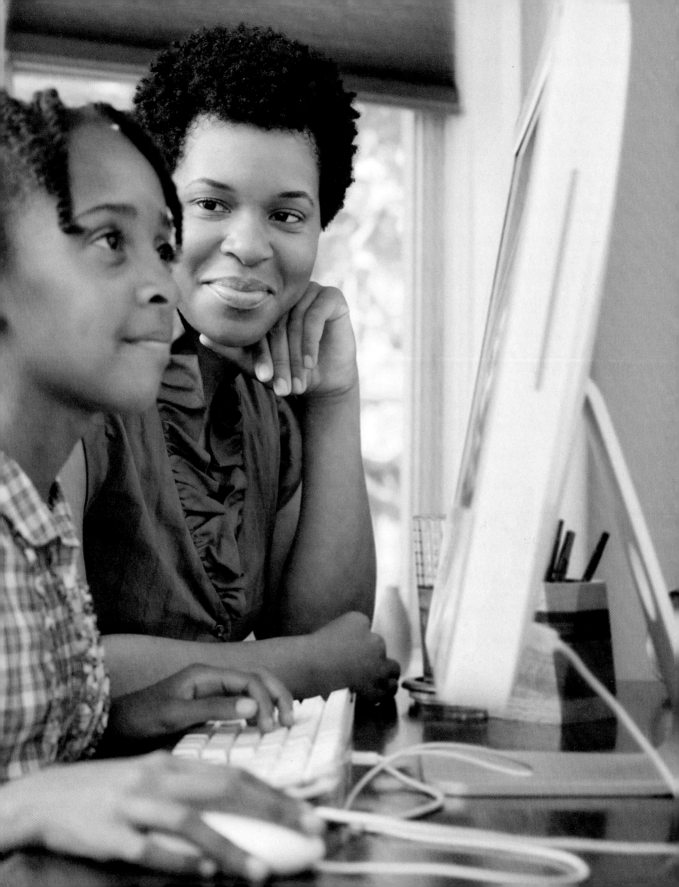

In an effort to portray a cool, sexy image, many adolescents post pictures similar to those that they see in the media. Suggestive poses or shots that feature kissing or other intimate acts are common—so common that to an adolescent mind, these pictures often do not cross any moral or social boundaries. They are simply a way of fitting in with friends and peers.

To monitor pictures and messages, you might consider becoming your child's "friend" on these networking sites. An adult presence may inhibit inappropriate or unsafe behavior. With an older teen, another option is to allow a private personal profile, with the understanding that you can have access to the account at any time.

Monitoring cell phones

Cell phones have increasing capabilities every year. Many now allow easy Internet access and have the capacity to send video or picture messages. These open up an ever-widening opportunity for your child to access or even create explicit, unmonitored content in a realm that often feels less sensored and more private than other technology tools.

Fortunately, checking in on your child's cell phone and texting habits is as easy as checking your phone bill. Your bill will tell you exactly which numbers your child is texting, and how often. Talk to your child if you notice excessive texts to an unfamiliar number. Checking your child's phone periodically is also an option, although this may not be as informative since texts and images can be deleted as soon as they are sent or received.

If you have concerns about texting habits, based on what you notice on your bill or simply on the amount of time your child spends texting, try saying something such as: "I was looking over our phone bill the other day, and noticed quite a lot of texts going from your phone to a number I didn't recognize. Can you tell me who this person is, and why you're texting so often?"

>>> YOUR CHILD MIGHT BE TARGETED BY AN ONLINE PREDATOR IF . . .

Online sexual predators come in many different shapes and sizes. Some pose as younger kids and create fake online identities in order to lure adolescents into trusting them. They might pretend to be from your child's school, or to have the same acquaintances. Predators adopt the language and demeanor of a sympathetic listener in order to gain trust. Your child might be at risk if he is:

• Spending increasing amounts of time online
• Spending much less time online, or acting nervous about the Internet
• Minimizing emails or chat sessions when you walk into the room
• Receiving frequent emails from someone you don't know
• Receiving phone calls or mail from someone you don't know
• Finding unusual or excessive spam in your inbox or your child's inbox
• Acting secretive about online activity
• Becoming unusually withdrawn from family and friends
• Acting sad or anxious, particularly after being online
• Spending less time with friends

"Sexting" and risk

Explicit activity via computer and cell phone has become so common that there is even a new word for it in our social lexicon. "Sexting" means to send or receive sexually explicit messages, pictures, or videos. A recent survey hosted by Teenage Research Unlimited found that 20% of teenagers in the United States have sexted using nude or semi-nude pictures.

Particularly when linked to the Internet, the possible repercussions of these photos and messages are tremendous. The original poster or sender loses control of the content once it appears online, so not only is this photo or video likely to be passed around the school, it is also likely to be passed around the web—possibly for many years to come. From college admission boards to future employers, anyone can potentially have immediate access to these ill-advised photo sessions.

Surprisingly, most teenagers are well aware of these consequences. 73% of teenagers in the Teenage Research Unlimited survey said they knew that posting or sending explicit photos could have "serious negative consequences." Still, many teens choose to take part in this trend. The truth is that until teens experience the negative results of sexting for themselves, the lesson might not hit home. An adolescent's intrinsic feelings of invincibility make learning from other people's bad decisions difficult. Add to that a teen's still-developing mind and judgment system, and it is no wonder that some teenagers don't see the harm in sexting.

While there is currently no research that shows that teens who engage in sexting are more likely to engage in sexual activity in real life, interacting with these messages repeatedly may desensitize teens and lead them to devalue their sexuality. The earlier a teen starts to explore sexuality with his peers, the harder it will be for him to make smart sexual decisions.

SEXPLANATION
WHAT DO POPULAR INTERNET ACRONYMS MEAN?

For adolescents, a big part of online culture is using the current code language. Some of these terms are innocent, and some are surprisingly explicit. Like all slang, these terms evolve frequently, so it's a good idea to stay educated on what the current codes mean.

ACRONYM	MEANING
GF	Girlfriend
BF	Boyfriend
BFF	Best friend forever
BRB	Be right back
AFK	Away from keyboard
BAK	Back at keyboard
CD9	Code 9—parents are around
PIR	Parent in room
PRW	Parents are watching (also PAW)
POS	Parent over shoulder
DOS	Dad over shoulder
MOS	Mom over shoulder
ILY	I love you
143	I love you
182	I hate you
ASL	Age/sex/location
LMIRL	Let's meet in real life
RU/18	Are you over 18?
KPC	Keeping parents clueless
KFY	Kiss for you (also K4Y)
BANANA	Penis
RUH	Are you horny?
DUM	Do you masturbate?
8	Oral sex
MEZRU	I am easy, are you?
IWSN	I want sex now
TDTM	Talk dirty to me
GNOC	Get naked on camera
GYPO	Get your pants off
NIFOC	Nude in front of the computer
FB	F*** buddy

Learning together

LEARNING ABOUT BEING SAFE ONLINE

The Internet is an invaluable tool and a useful source of information and entertainment for children. It is important to help your child make the most of what it has to offer while staying safe online. You don't have to be a computer expert to teach your child how to protect himself—most of what he needs to know is based on common sense. As early as 5 or 6, begin checking that your child is aware of all the potential dangers. Try to agree on a code of conduct to be followed whenever he goes online.

AFTER THIS LESSON YOUR CHILD WILL BE MORE LIKELY TO...
- Understand the potential risks involved in going online
- Keep his personal details, and those of his family and friends, to himself
- Be aware that people in chat rooms may not be who they seem
- Use online networking responsibly
- Ask you before agreeing to meet anyone he has chatted with online
- Tell you if he feels uncomfortable about anything that happens online

1 WHAT ARE THE RISKS ONLINE?

Try having this conversation when your child is at the computer. Sit down next to him and show an interest in what he is doing. Ask him first what he likes best about using the Internet. Then ask if he knows the difference between editorial content and advertising, and look for examples to illustrate both. Next, steer the chat toward potential dangers he might encounter online. Possible questions to ask include: Does he realize that the people he meets in chat rooms might not always be as they seem? What does he imagine might happen if he gave out his phone number, address, or email to a stranger? What might be the consequences of giving out personal information or family or friends' details on a social networking site? What would he do if someone he didn't know asked to meet him in person? When he searches the web for information, how does he distinguish fact from fiction? These types of questions will help you establish how net-wise your child really is, and will also help him think through the possible consequences of careless online decisions and actions.

2 HOW CAN CHILDREN PROTECT THEMSELVES?

The golden rule for all online activities is that your child should never reveal personal information without your consent. Let your child know that websites often ask for personal details in order to take part in competitions or offers, and that your child should always check with you first, even if the site is run by an organization he knows. You can also take this opportunity to talk about the way some people behave in chat rooms. Remind your child to be very careful about people online who offer easy solutions to difficult problems or make offers that seem too good to be true. Tell your child that it's best not to open emails from strangers. If he does inadvertently open mail, he should not click on any links, open attachments, or take any action without first checking with you. Similarly, he should not send or post any photos of himself without talking to you first.

3 HOW SHOULD THE NASTY STUFF BE DEALT WITH?

Explain to your child that while much of the content online is useful, entertaining, and positive, there is also material that is obscene, highly offensive, cruel, or hateful, and that should be avoided at all costs. While filtering programs can protect your children to a large extent while they are young, these technologies are not the complete answer, as some harmful content is presented in subtle forms that are not caught by filters. Educate older children to surf uncensored online territory sensibly and in accordance with their family values. Point out that the difference between right and wrong is the same on the Internet as it is in real life. Make your child aware of the existence of sites and groups that encourage cruelty or racial hatred. Often the purpose of these sites is not always immediately obvious. Some even encourage children by offering what seem like harmless activities to draw them in. If a web site looks suspicious or has a warning page for people under 18 years of age, your child should exit it immediately.

4   WHAT IS CYBER BULLYING?

Explain to your child that "cyber bullying" is the term used to describe any kind of online intimidation, such as receiving unwanted or nasty emails or having something posted on a website about you. If your child ever receives an inappropriate or disturbing email from someone he thinks he knows, such as someone at school, tell him not to reply. The sender is looking for a reaction, just as he or she would if bullying your child in person. The best way to encourage online bullies to stop is to not give them the satisfaction of replying. Let your child know that if the bully doesn't stop, you will help find out where the emails are coming from and contact the school or service provider as appropriate. If bullying is taking place on a school or community website, stress to your child that he should do exactly as he would as if he were being bullied face to face—and tell either you or a teacher about it.

5   HOW CAN STAYING SAFE BE ENCOURAGED?

Children need to learn how to look after themselves and make wise decisions online, just as they do in the real world. Encourage your child to take responsibility for his own safety, though at the same time he needs to feel able to come to you with any concerns or worries. Ask your child if he—or anyone he knows—has ever encountered anything inappropriate or frightening online. If your child confides in you, try not to overreact, blame your child, or take away Internet privileges, as this may discourage him from being open with you in the future. Instead, be supportive and decide how to best prevent the problem from repeating itself. Teach your child to end any experience online immediately if he feels uncomfortable, and to tell you or another trusted adult in these cases.

HOW TO ANSWER QUESTIONS ABOUT SAFETY ONLINE

Try to get to know the Internet services your child uses so that you can answer any questions he might have. You can also have your child show you what he does online. Encourage your child to ask questions, and If you don't know the answer to something, tell your child that you will find out. Then, speak to another adult who uses the Internet often, or visit your library for information.

Q. Is information that I share online private?
A. Few things on the Internet are truly private. Words or pictures that are shared online will often be brought up when someone searches for your name.

Q. How can you identify an online predator?
A. This is hard. Predators can be very clever in the way they establish relationships. Be vigilant at all times, and tell an adult immediately if anyone tries to introduce sexual content into any conversation.

Learning together

Encouraging positive media influences

Equally important as protecting your child against negative media influences is remembering that not all media tears down. Some media builds up, and can even help guide and instruct your child. A good approach is to promote positive media outlets, stay connected to current popular culture and media trends, and allow your child just enough space to develop personal tastes and interests.

Staying connected to pop culture

Understanding the cultural influences that are part of your child's world is a must for involved parents. The best way to do this is to simply stay aware and interested in your child's world. Watch, read, and listen to popular programming, music, and literature, and ask your child to introduce you to the things that he is interested in. Adolescence is probably the first time that your child will try to define what he listens to, what he watches, and what he reads. Allow his natural curiosity and self-expression to develop, so long as you don't notice anything destructive in his choices. This small freedom can help foster trust in your relationship and also show your child that you are interested in his own personal taste and style.

The next time you go on a road trip together, don't maintain strict control of the stereo. Let your child choose the music, and assimilate a little bit into the world he is growing up in. The more attuned you are to the media influences in your child's life, the better you will be able to understand the environment he is growing up in. Not only will this give you common ground and conversation topics, it will also help you understand his point-of-view and offer him the support and patience he needs as he grows. In addition, showing interest in his world can be hugely nurturing to his self-esteem.

Promoting positive media outlets

You can contribute to your child's interests by presenting her with positive media influences, perhaps ones that you enjoyed as a child. This is a good way both to share your interests and to direct the type of media content she sees. Movies, books, and music that celebrate love—not just sex—can be especially effective at encouraging your child to make decisions based on values, not physical temptation.

Create a weekly movie night tradition where you spend one week watching a classic movie of your choice and the next week watching a contemporary movie that your child chooses. This allows you to monitor her interests and ensure that her choices are age-appropriate. It is equally good for helping you understand each other better, and learning to see each other as individuals with unique interests and tastes, rather than simply as "parent" and "child."

You can also stress positive media influences by giving your child a book you enjoyed at her age, or introducing her to an author whose books have influenced you. Talk about the book together as your child reads it, and recall your own feelings and thoughts that you had when you were younger. You can then encourage your child to share a book or author that she loves, or to show you her favorite magazines and explain why she likes them or identifies with them.

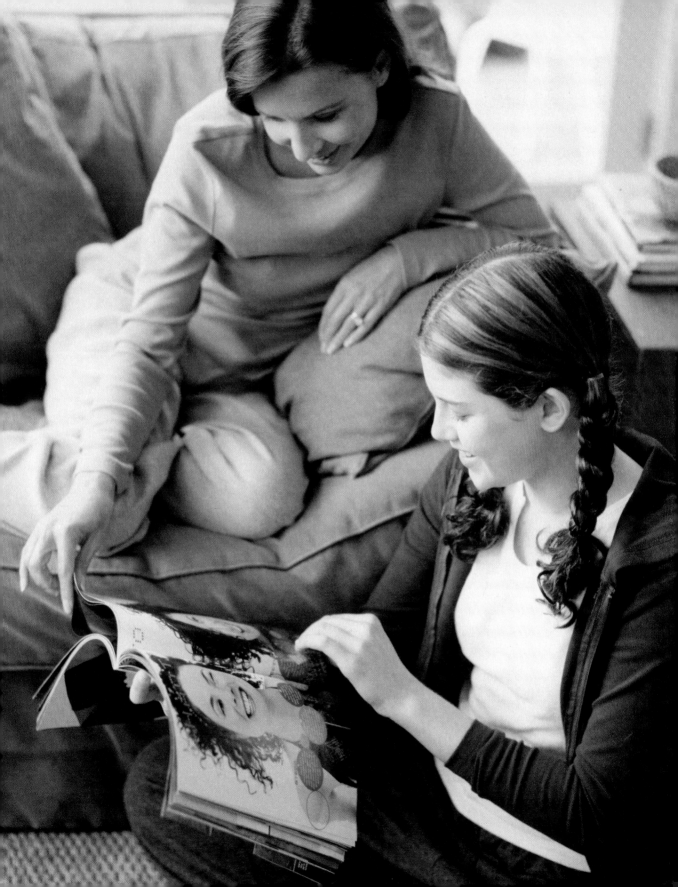

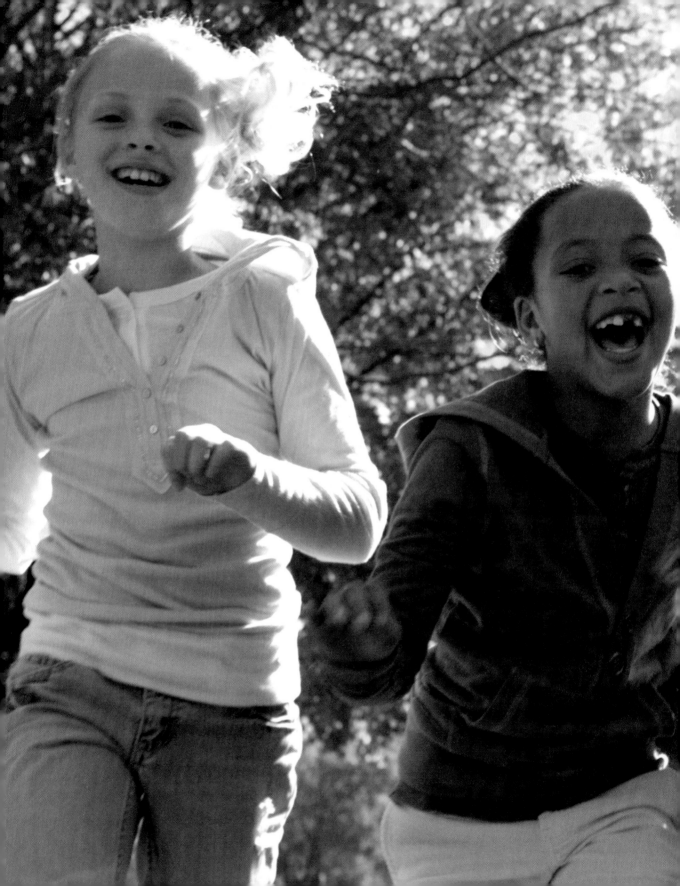

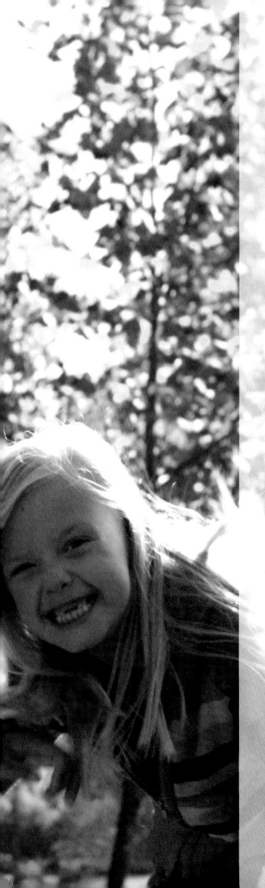

4

TALKING ABOUT FRIENDS AND INFLUENCES

ASSESSING YOUR VALUES: FRIENDS AND INFLUENCES

While you can't decide who your child becomes friends with, you can help monitor his social circle and the people who impact him. The first step to being a positive influence is to determine what family rules and guidelines you want to establish about friendship and social activities. The second is to analyze how your own friendships can set a good example. Reflect on these questions individually, then talk with your partner about the best way to guide this important part of your child's identity.

EXPLORING FRIENDSHIP

Thinking about what qualities are important to you in a friend will help ensure that you proactively pass along this important message to your child. This can help encourage positive friendships and, down the road, can also help encourage positive romantic relationships.

• What qualities are valuable to you in a friend?

• What types of friendships are important to you?

• Do you have close friendships? Have you maintained your friendships over the years?

• What lessons—consciously or subconsciously—have you taught your child about friendship?

• Do you live a social lifestyle, or do you and your partner tend to spend time primarily with each other and with your kids?

• Are you close with your siblings and other family members? Does your child have a tight-knit family around him?

• Have your friendships changed dramatically over the years? Do you still have close friends that you've know since childhood?

• Are most of your friends of the same gender?

EXPLORING SOCIAL INVOLVEMENT

Staying involved in your child's social life is the best way to monitor her development and behavior, and can help protect her from negative influences. It is a good idea to plan ahead of time about what type of involvement you want to have.

• How involved are you in your child's social world, including life at school and involvement in extracurricular activities?

• How aware are you of trends/activities/lifestyle choices for your child's age group?

• How can you encourage your child to make new friends, and to be confident reaching out to others in new social situations?

• What social activities do you think are important to monitor?

• How do you develop and maintain a sense of trust in the parent/child relationship?

• What will you do if you find out that your child is being bullied at school?

• What will you do if he is the bully?

• How do you encourage your child's independence, if at all?

- How well do you know your child's friends?

- How involved are you in your child's friends' lives? Do you know their parents, where they live, their likes/dislikes, etc.?

EXPLORING SOCIAL RULES

Determining family rules about friendship and social activities from an early age can help ensure your child grows up sharing and respecting important values, and will also help you stay conscious of establishing a positive home environment.

- What rules do you think should be in place when your child has friends over (e.g. bedroom door open, parent always home, etc.)?

- What consequences do you think should exist for breaking those rules?

- Do you think different rules should exist for friendships with members of the opposite sex?

- What actions would you want to take if your child makes friends you don't trust or don't deem appropriate?

- How much time do you think your child should devote to nourishing friendships (e.g. as much as he likes, as much as he can while still doing well in school, etc.)?

- How much freedom will you allow your child as he gets older?

- At what age do you think it's appropriate for your child to make his own decisions about friends, curfew, parties, etc.?

- How important do you think it is for your child's friends to come from families with similar rules and expectations around social activities?

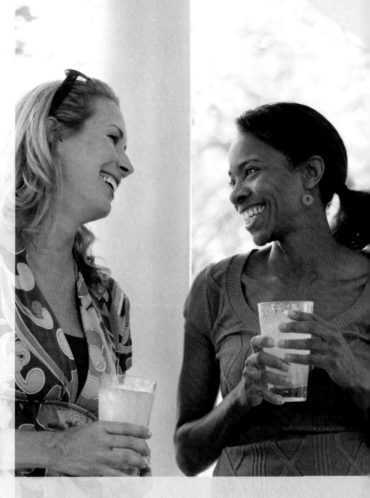

APPLYING YOUR ANSWERS Friendships are something we often think should happen naturally, but the truth is that you can purposefully decide what types of people you want in your life—and help your child to make these positive decisions, too. If you and your partner have different views on friendship, that's okay. What is important is establishing friendship as a vital part of health and happiness. If you can agree on the qualities that make a good friend and on how involved you want to be in your child's social world, you are ready to begin this part of your child's education.

Your child's social development

To help establish a healthy social setting for your child, you first must understand the day-to-day realities he faces. Although development differs for every child, there are established stages that can help prepare you for how your child will see and interact with the world. In addition, these stages can signal when he will become more aware of and interested in sexual relationships.

Stages of social development

Created by psychiatrist Erik Erikson in 1956, the Stages of Social Development illustrate how social awareness grows. Of course, every child matures differently depending on a variety of factors. Children might also progress or regress unexpectedly. However, knowing these stages can help you learn how to relate to your child about feelings, friends, and developing sexuality.

Trust vs. mistrust, 0–2 years: A child learns trust or mistrust based on the behavior of her caretakers. If a child is well cared for, and is regularly fed, bathed, and cuddled, she will learn a basic sense of trust. If not, she will develop a sense of mistrust, which might exhibit itself later in life as anxiety or suspicion.

Social interaction varies during this stage. Until a child is about one year old, she will only interact with adults through actions like smiling and cooing. When your child is between 1 and 1½ years old, she will enjoy solitary play. At this point, she will only play alone, although she may want an adult to watch or encourage her play.

Autonomy vs. shame, 2–4 years: Your child is beginning to walk and talk like the adults around him. He has developed a sense of self and craves more autonomy, which may lead to temper tantrums, a.k.a. the "terrible twos."

If a child is supported and encouraged during this time, he will develop confidence. If his parents are anxious or overly protective, the child might develop feelings of shame or self-doubt. At this developing age, encouraging him to be open about his body is especially important, and can help ensure that he doesn't experience feelings of shame or guilt about his body or sexuality in later life.

Socially speaking, a child between the ages of 2–2 ½ begins to engage in "parallel play," which means that he will begin to enjoy playing alongside other children. This play will rarely involve much sharing of toys or interaction—children will simply begin to enjoy sitting alongside each other (hence the term "parallel").

Initiative vs. guilt, 3–5 years: At this age, most children are learning basic lessons like reading and writing. As a result, they might start to develop purpose, as well as active imaginations and interest in new activities. Some children, however, do not want to venture out so readily into this new world, and instead cling to their parents or other adults. Between these ages, children also experience their first feelings of guilt and frustration, perhaps from being unable to complete a puzzle or read or pronounce a word. Additionally, sexual guilt may begin if a child is reprimanded or made to feel ashamed or embarrassed about her body.

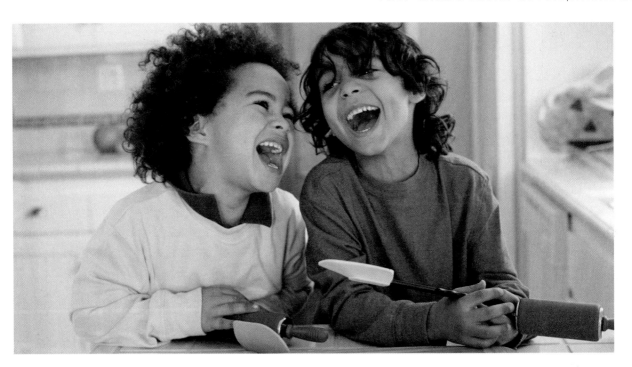

Starting around 3 years of age, a child's social interaction develops so that she begins to enjoy engaging in activities with other children, such as singing or coloring. However, children of this age don't actually play cooperatively with other children, as they are still in an ego-centric stage.

Industry vs. inferiority, 5–12 years: Throughout these years, a child will develop a stronger sense of identity and will also begin to form moral values. A child who has developed securely throughout each of the past social stages will be successful and confident, whereas a child who has struggled through the earlier stages might suffer from feelings of self-doubt or inferiority. These anxieties can lead to poor body image, early sexual insecurity, and difficulty making friends and fitting in with their peers.

Social interaction develops hugely during this period. Starting around 4 or 5 years of age, your child will begin to play cooperatively. She will be able to take turns, follow directions, and work for a common goal with a team or a group. During this time, your child will enter into real social interaction that is not ego-centric, but is based on the needs and interests of others.

Identity vs. role confusion, 12–21 years: During this time, adolescents seek to answer life's most important question: "Who am I?" Your child might experiment with different roles, and perhaps with behavior that you consider risky, such as drinking or experimenting with various sexual partners. He will also seek mentors and outside influences in an attempt to form his own identity. The way he is viewed by his peers becomes very important during this stage.

During the later years, your child will also develop his sexual identity, and come to terms with his sexual desires. Exploring sexual identity will include exploring new roles within that identity, such as boyfriend or lover. Your child will seek to know what these roles mean and whether he is successful at them.

Getting to know your child's friends

Knowing and being liked by your child's friends can play a huge role in the closeness of your relationship with your child. Make it a point to encourage positive activities, entertain your child's friends at home, and help foster a vital, secure community for your child. A healthy home environment that overlaps with your child's social group can protect against unsafe sexual behavior and other risks.

Encouraging healthy involvement

As a parent, you can have a very hands-on role in creating your child's social circle, and also in helping him develop certain social behaviors. This does not meant that you need to be smothering. Encouraging your child to participate in activities such as sports teams, dance classes, acting troupes, summer camps, and church youth groups makes it more likely that he will be part of a positive social environment. While it is a good idea not to overextend your child by scheduling every moment of the day, encouraging him to choose just one or two social groups outside of school can help him form a variety of friendships and interests, which in turn will help foster a healthy self-esteem and strong identity.

Additionally, it is a good idea to encourage your child to stay connected at school. Teens who are involved in school activities and school functions, regardless of the activity, are less likely to take sexual risks and likely to postpone sex. Greater involvement in school is also linked to decreased teen pregnancy rates.

Getting to know your child's friends

Getting to know your child's friends can be daunting, especially during the teenage years. You might think, "I barely know my own teenager, how can I get to know a whole group of them?" Luckily, it isn't as difficult as it sounds, though it might take some patience and sacrifice on your part. A good way to start is to keep the house stocked with snacks and allow your child freedom to play and socialize at home. This way, your child and her friends will be more likely to spend time in the safety of your own house and you will have a better opportunity to keep an eye on your child, get to know her friends, and monitor her activities and influences.

As an active participant in your child's social circle, you can spend more time talking to your child's friends. Having these close relationships is important because it helps you stay connected to your child, gives you a greater level of insight into her social world, and keeps you informed of any negative influences that might encourage inappropriate or premature sexual behavior. Understanding these influences can help you combat them, and will also give you a chance to answer any questions your child might have. For example, if you know that your child's friend has an older sister who is pregnant, you can talk about this with your child and help her to understand and process the situation.

You might say something like: "Your friend Billy told me last night that his sister is pregnant. She just turned 15 years old. Do you know her? How do you feel about what has happened? Does Billy have any questions or concerns about it?"

Your influence

Apart from helping foster a positive social environment, your own social habits will play a role in creating your child's social behaviors. Children naturally watch the way their parents interact with the outside world, and often mimic those behaviors. If you are an open person, your child might develop this openness, too. If you are closed off from others, your child might pick up on any reticence or a sense of mistrust.

Your child will also notice how much time you spend on your own friendships and interests. Many parents do not have a strong social circle. The demands of parenthood, along with work and other responsibilities, often leave little time for friendships. However, this can be harmful to your own quality of life, as well as to your child's social outlook. It is important for your child to see you as a social, active adult, who develops personal interests and maintains personal friendships. Whether this means being active in your church or having a weekly workout date with your next door neighbor, maintaining a happy social life should not be seen as selfish or as taking time away from your child. Instead, you are giving your child a great gift—the image of a happy, fulfilled adult with successful, long-lasting social bonds.

Having an active social life can also help create a loving and supportive community for your child, especially if you live far away from your relatives or if you have a small family. Try getting involved in your church or synagogue, volunteering at a senior center, hosting a block party, gettin involved in school activities, or simply becoming friendly with the parents of your child's peers, perhaps at the park or at PTA meetings. Establishing a variety of friends is a good way to help develop your child's own social circle. This can also ensure that your child has strong, positive adult role models in his life outside of you and your partner.

WHAT TO SAY. . .
IF YOU THINK YOUR CHILD IS HAVING TROUBLE MAKING FRIENDS:

As a parent, it is incredibly painful to see your child lonely or rejected by peers. Choose a time during the weekend, when your child won't be worried about school, to start a conversation about this.

CONVERSATION STARTER: "I have noticed recently that you and [insert friend's name] don't seem as close anymore. Do you feel like that is true?"

Allow your child a chance to respond, and look to see if he seems hurt or sad when talking about this particular friend. You can then ask him more directly about the relationship.

FOLLOW-UP: "Do you miss [name of friend]? Did anything happen between the two of you to damage or change your friendship?"

Once your child has had a chance to talk about the relationship, you can empathize with him and also share a positive anecdote.

FOLLOW-UP: "I remember a time when I was younger and kids at school weren't very welcoming. I wanted to run away and never go back, but instead, I joined the soccer team."

Ask your child if there are any new activities that he thinks sound fun, or that he is interested in joining. Sometimes a change in environment or involvement can provide a significant self-esteem boost, and also help get your child's mind off any worries or painful experiences with friends.

FOLLOW-UP: "I made so many new friends on the team. And once the other kids saw that I was open to making new friends, they became more friendly. Remember that there are a lot of kids out there who want friends, especially a good friend like you."

Friends and sexual influences

Friends hold huge sway over your child's sexual decisions, especially during the teenage years when the emphasis is on growing up as fast as possible. While you can't entirely monitor the sexual influences your teenager will encounter everyday, you can stay aware of behavioral patterns and social pressures.

Friends and sexual activity

A recent study performed at the University of Minnesota found that a child's social circle has a significant impact on that child's likelihood to engage in intercourse. In the study, it was found that adolescents who had more sexually experienced friends were much more likely to become sexually active themselves. These odds were even higher in cases where adolescents believed that sexual activity would help them earn greater respect from their friends.

Of course, it might be argued that teens that are more open to sexual activity are also more likely to be friends with teens who are sexually active. Either way, it is clear that the behavior of your child's social circle is a good indicator of your child's own behavior. In fact, similar research has found that adolescents who have friends who are abstinent tend to have equally strong feelings about abstinence. Thus, a child who is surrounded by friends that provide a positive sexual influence will find it much more easy to abstain from sex.

Analyzing your child's behavior

Even the most involved parents sometimes find themselves unaware of their child's activities, especially as he grows older. This can be true even if your child is fairly open and you have a close relationship. As much as possible, pay close attention to your child's actions and look for any changes in behavior that might indicate

>>> **YOUR CHILD MIGHT BE EXPOSED TO NEGATIVE PEER PRESSURE IF . . .**

When your child is being affected by negative influences, behavioral changes are usually the first sign. She might generally seem anxious, frustrated, or even unexpectedly guilty. If you notice these symptoms in addition to the more specific signs below, it is a good idea to talk with your child about whether she is happy in her current social environment.

• Developing a different manner of dress or speech
• Hanging out with a new crowd of friends that you don't know
• Seeming withdrawn or not wanting to spend time with old friends
• A drop in grades or a disinterest in favorite activities
• Being very secretive about her whereabouts and behavior outside the home

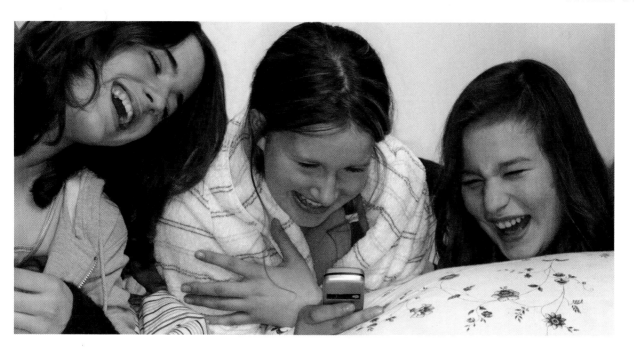

that he is affected by new and possibly risky influences. Signs of this can include changes in personality or in the level of involvement and interest in family activities.

One cause for concern may be if your child is spending time solely with a new group of friends. While it is natural for a teen to explore different social circles as he searches for his own identity, be aware of a situation in which he completely abandons all of his former friends and acquaintances. A completely new set of friends might mean that your child is moving onto new activities that his old friends might not approve of or enjoy. This is especially true if your child's wardrobe changes dramatically at the same time, or if there are other outward signs of a change in perspective or interests. If you notice an abrupt change in your child's group of friends, tune into this warning sign and ask him about it.

You might say something like "What ever happened to Brian and Daniel? Do you still talk to Kevin? I haven't seen those guys in a while."

Similarly, pay attention to the words your child is using. Parents often tend to tune out when teens are on the phone, but by simply listening to your child's conversations, you can pick up on social clues. If it appears that your teen is speaking in code, or if he becomes very upset if his phone privacy is interrupted in any way, he may be talking about something that is inappropriate or even explicit. Have an honest talk with him about behavior that concerns you and if it continues, consider taking him to a family or adolescent counselor.

Also watch for an obsession with chewing gum, mouthwash, body spray, or other tools that disguise scent. Of course, all of these are normal to use in moderation, but if your child carries these things with him at all times, it might be a sign that he is trying to hide something. Constant use might signal an attempt to mask the smell of alcohol or smoke—influences which can severely hinder judgment, and in turn can suggest that your child is at greater risk of engaging in inappropriate sexual activity.

Learning together

LEARNING ABOUT NEGATIVE PEER PRESSURE

No influence in your teenager's life is as powerful as peer pressure. At its best, it can motivate your child and boost her self-esteem, at its worst, it can impair good judgment and lead her into dangerous activities, including sex. Help your child to cope with negative peer pressure by encouraging her to think independently and make her own decisions. Around the ages of 8 or 9, before negative peer pressure becomes a serious threat, discuss the best ways of overcoming this obstacle to happiness.

AFTER THIS LESSON YOUR CHILD WILL BE MORE LIKELY TO...
- Know who her peers are and the kinds of pressure she is likely to face
- Understand that she does not always have to hang out with the "in" crowd
- Realize the importance of making her own decisions and judgments
- Resist the pressure to have sex, take drugs, or engage in any type of risky behavior or activities
- Know that you are on her side and will help her if she needs it.

1 WHAT IS PEER PRESSURE?
Explain to your child that a big part of growing older is making challenging decisions. These decisions can involve serious moral questions, like should you skip class or go further than just kissing? Point out that making these types of decisions on your own is tough, but that it can be even harder when people your own age (your peers) get involved and try to influence you one way or the other. Peer pressure is something that everyone has to handle, even adults, and it can be difficult to deal with because we all want to be liked. Point out that peer pressure isn't always negative; good friends can encourage you to do positive things, too. It becomes a problem if it results in you risking your safety or compromising your values.

2 WHAT ARE THE BEST WAYS OF DEALING WITH OR MINIMIZING PEER PRESSURE?
Ask your child how she would feel about saying "no" to her friends. Explain that it takes courage to say "no," but that it's better than finding herself in a situation she does not want to be in. Encourage her to follow her instincts and beliefs about what is right and wrong to help her know what to do. Talk about the kinds of pressure she might be subjected to. What would she do if her friends tried to persuade her to drink alcohol? Try role-playing if you think this would help your teen frame a response she feels happy with. Also let her know that it's fine to blame you by saying something like, "No thanks—If Mom or Dad smells smoke on me, I'll be grounded for weeks."

3 HOW DO YOU COPE WITH PEER PRESSURE TO BECOME SEXUALLY ACTIVE?
Both boys and girls often feel enormous pressure to have sex—or to engage in sexual activities—before they are ready. To help counteract this, explain that lots of teenagers regret having sex too early. Try to convince your teen how important it is to be strong and stand up for what she feels is right. Encourage her to think about how she would respond if pressured to have sex. If someone says, "Everyone is doing it," for example, she could respond by saying "I'm my own person—I don't have to do something because everyone else does." If it is your child's boyfriend or girlfriend who is applying pressure, troubleshooting how to respond to statements like, "If you really loved me you would have sex," may help your child identify these as a form of manipulation.

Any kind of coercion, particularly when it comes to sex, is not a sign of a healthy relationship, and your child should reconsider its standing. Tell your child that a significant other who really cared would respect her wish not to rush into sex. Teens who want to defend their reasons for not having sex could say something like, "I don't want to risk getting (you) pregnant" or "I want to wait until I'm married."

4 IN WHAT WAYS DOES PEER PRESSURE AFFECT BODY IMAGE?

The chances are high that your child has felt pressure from peers to look a certain way. Talk to your child about the pressure to fit physical ideals, which can be particularly tough for those who don't quite fit the "cool" image. Most children get their ideas of what is desirable from television and magazines. Yet celebrities and models are rarely what they seem. Point out to your child that pictures of male and female models portrayed in magazines are altered with airbrushing and fancy lighting. Explain that the images tend not to reflect different shapes, cultures, and sizes, much less personality, character, sense of humor, compassion, or intelligence—all the qualities that really define a person. Try to instill in your child that self-worth comes from within, not from how you look on the outside. Stress that your child doesn't have to listen to what other people say about her appearance, and that she has the right to be happy just as she is.

5 WHAT IF YOU GIVE IN TO PEER PRESSURE?

Let your child know that everyone makes mistakes—it's part of growing up. Say that you understand the kinds of pressures she faces and realize how difficult it can be to resist that pressure. Stress how proud you are of her and of her accomplishments. Most teenagers succumb to peer pressure at some point, so your child should not feel overly guilty, although she should understand the consequences that can result from her decisions. Explain that the most important thing is to learn from the experience and try to come up with a better solution for the next time such a situation arises. Reassure your child that she can call you to come and pick her up or get her out of a difficult situation at any time. You can also explain that it's fine to distance herself from friends or classmates who are critical, and to seek out new relationships that are more positive. Above all, let your child know that if she needs help or guidance at any time, you are there for her.

HOW TO ANSWER QUESTIONS ABOUT NEGATIVE PEER PRESSURE

Try to recognize that fitting in with a peer group is very serious and important to your teenager. Use questions as opportunities for discussion about situations and incidents without being judgmental or punitive. This will encourage your teenager to trust you for advice about the specific issues that she is facing.

Q. What if all my friends are drinking at a party?
A. Remember the reasons why drinking can be dangerous, and simply say that you choose not to drink. Surprisingly, though it may seem like you have to drink to fit in, most teens won't mention it again once you verbalize your decision.

Q. What if my date asks me to go to a new level physically?
A. Say "no" to anything that makes you uncomfortable or compromises your values. If your date cannot accept your answer, he is not a good person to begin a relationship with.

Learning together

Monitoring activities

Part of being a parent means walking a fine line between staying involved and giving your child space to explore. Too little supervision can cause your child to feel unloved and can pave the way for unsafe behavior. Too much, and your child may become frustrated and rebel. The trick is finding a balance that gives your child both a sense of freedom and a sense of responsibility.

Setting and enforcing rules

The first step in setting household rules that will be followed is to find discipline tactics that both you and your partner can uphold at all times. A punishment that is rarely enforced won't have much effect on your child—and worse, when it is enforced, it may seem unfair. A clear set of rules and consequences will ensure that your child understands what she needs to do in order to uphold family values and expectations.

Try not to discipline in anger. While it is okay to let your child know that you are angry with him, it is also important to retain control over your emotions. Take a few moments to cool down so you can think and speak clearly. This can also teach your child to grow into a rational adult who doesn't give in to angry impulses.

Avoid criticism. There is a big difference between criticism and negative feedback—criticism can cut your child down, while negative feedback allows your child to be proactive about changing behavior. For example, if your child didn't take out the trash as promised, and you lash out and say "I can't believe you didn't clean your room again! You are so ungrateful and spoiled!" your child will feel hurt and angry. However, if you say, "I see you didn't pick up your room like I asked. When you do that, it hurts my feelings because it makes me feel like you aren't listening to me and you don't appreciate all the things I do for you," your child will be more likely to understand where you are coming from, and also to see a clear plan of action he needs to follow in the future.

Adjusting rules

Specific rules and consequences will change as your child grows older and can handle more responsibility. You can encourage positive behavior by allowing your child more freedom every time he shows good judgement. For example, if your child is honest about something he did wrong, reward him by showing more trust the next time he goes out with friends.

It is also a good idea to allow your child to make his own decisions sometimes, so that he can learn to trust his judgment. For example, if you know he is going to spend his allowance on the hot new electronic toy, don't try to stop him—but also remind him of his choice when he wants more money later in the month. Setting up small situations like this where your child can learn from mistakes will help him learn to make smart decisions, both sexually and otherwise. The goal of discipline is to teach your child positive values so that he will grow into a capable adult. Without some freedom to make his own small mistakes, he won't learn these valuable lessons until later in life—at which time his mistakes might not be so small.

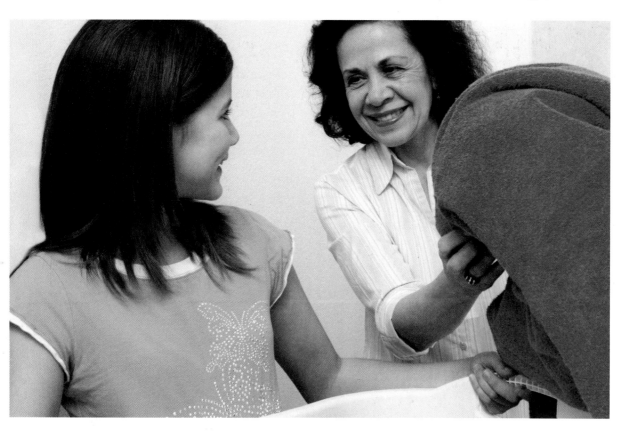

TEACHABLE MOMENT
TALKING ABOUT UNSAFE ACTIVITIES

The next time you and your child are paging through celebrity magazines awash with the latest Hollywood scandals, make a note to use these incidents to spark a discussion. For example, you might say: "Did you see that magazine headline about the celebrity being arrested for a DUI? She's not that much older than you. Have any of your friends ever driven after drinking? How did that make you feel?" You can also use this moment to let your child know that if she is ever in a situation where she feels uncomfortable—whether it involves drinking, drugs, or sex—she can call you and you will instantly come pick her up, without asking any questions.

CONVERSATION STARTER 1: "I am glad that you have been making so many new friends lately. What do you usually do together? Remember that if you ever feel uneasy about any activity, you can always call and have me come pick you up. I won't ever judge you for the situation you find yourself in, and it is a very mature choice to remove yourself from anything that makes you uncomfortable."

CONVERSATION STARTER 2: "It seems like celebrities are getting caught using illegal drugs more and more. Are any kids in your school involved with that? Have you ever felt pressure to do drugs?"

Encouraging positive friendships

Teaching your child to recognize and pursue close friendships will help her develop a strong sense of self-esteem and encourage her to make other positive relationship decisions as she grows up. Children with supportive, close-knit groups of friends are less likely to become involved in a romantic or sexual relationship that is not equally supportive and fulfilling.

Teaching by example

Starting from a young age, it is important for your child to learn the basic values of friendship from you. For example, if your child is just starting to make friends and socialize with other children, make it a point to mention when your friend does something nice for you, such as "Did you see how my friend Sarah let me borrow her DVD? She is such a good friend, isn't she? Don't you like it when you and your friends share?"

Older children will understand ideas like sharing and kindness, but they are still learning how to treat friends. Because of this, it is important to try to avoid gossip and other hurtful behaviors. Instead, show your child how to communicate with his friends in a more respectful and open fashion.

For example, you might share: "I was angry with Sarah the other day for missing our lunch plans. I called her and told her how I felt about it, though, rather than gossiping about it. I knew it would hurt her feelings if I mentioned it to other people, and once I heard her side of the story, I realized she didn't miss our lunch intentionally."

It is also a good idea to show your child that your friends respect you in return. If he sees you being pushed around by friends, he might be more likely to adopt similar behavior in his own friendships. Instead, teach your child to be authentic with friends about his feelings and needs. This will help him learn how to maintain strong bonds and positive friendships. Growing up in an environment of positive relationships will help your child mirror these lessons both in friendships and in romantic relationships.

Talking about image vs. identity

As your child reaches adolescence, her main focus will be discovering her own identity. This can be a stressful and sometimes painful experience. You can help your child during this time by emphasizing that identity is not based on image, despite the messages she may hear from friends and the media. If your child doesn't believe that appearance and image are everything, her identity will be more deep-rooted and stable.

A good way to encourage this viewpoint from an early age is to refrain from making negative comments about people's appearances. When you make frequent comments about people's weight or appearance, your child will start to internalize those judgments, and will be more likely to begin judging herself and the people around her based on appearance.

In addition, make an effort to share positive comments with others and with your child. Try to underscore positive qualities that have nothing to do with how your child looks. This is especially important to remember when raising young girls. It can be a good self-esteem builder to pay appearance-based compliments, but be sure that you don't exclusively praise your daughter's appearance or she might grow up thinking that beauty is her most praise-worthy characteristic. Make it a point to tell her how funny she is, how smart she is, how strong she is, or what a good friend she is to others. By focusing on qualities other than appearance, you can help your child create an identity that has nothing to do with her weight or what she is wearing. In turn, she will be more likely to judge people based on their actions and character, and to choose friends that have similar values to hers. Instilling positive feedback and values in your child will help her make friends that you approve of and trust.

Encouraging the right friendships

While you cannot choose your child's friends for him, you can help him to choose friends that treat others well. Talk to your child from an early age about the importance of being friends with children who get along with others. With an older child, you might continue this influence by praising the things you like about his friends. The more you encourage your child to form bonds with people who exhibit positive behavior and self-confidence, the more he can learn from these behaviors.

For example, you might say: "I liked the friend you brought home for dinner yesterday. She seems very smart and motivated. I hope you bring her around more often."

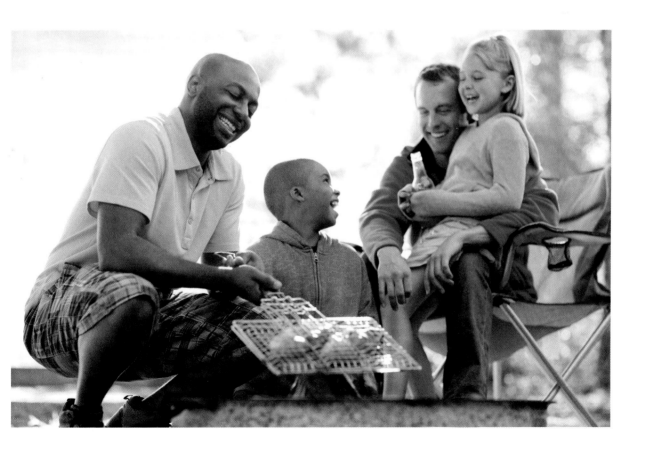

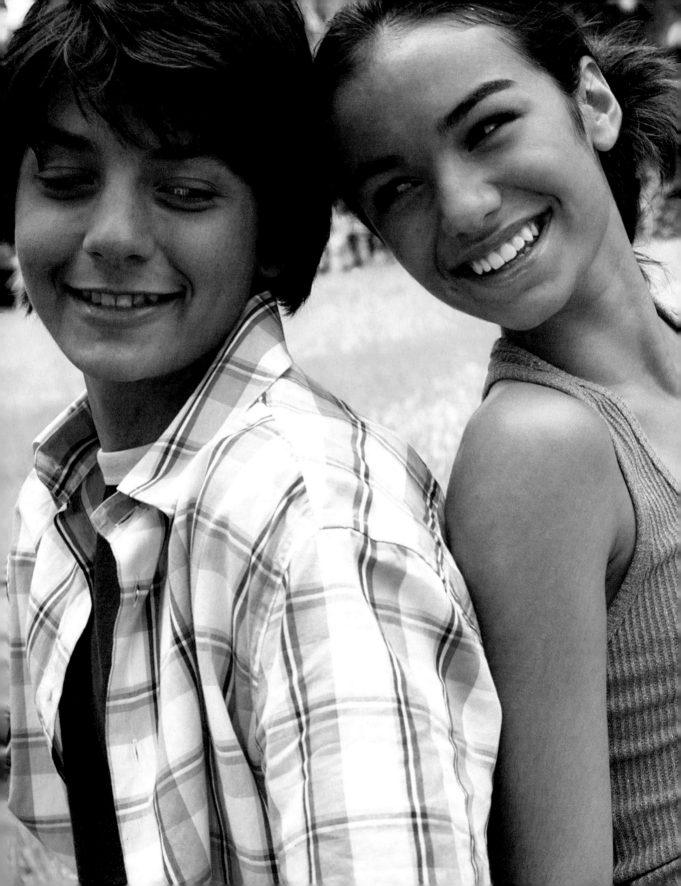

5

TALKING ABOUT ROMANTIC RELATIONSHIPS

ASSESSING YOUR VALUES: ROMANTIC RELATIONSHIPS

Your child's first romantic relationship is a milestone—both for your child and for you as a parent. It can also be a challenge to encourage and support your child as he begins to make relationship decisions. Thinking in advance about how you want to guide your child through this time can make help minimize any uncertainties you might have. Consider the following questions privately to help clarify your feelings, then discuss them with a partner.

EXPLORING RELATIONSHIP READINESS

Being ready to be in a relationship is more about maturity and character then about age. Thinking about the qualities that are important for a fulfilling relationship will help you better determine when your child has reached that point and is ready for that type of commitment.

• At what age do you think you should begin talking to your child about relationships?

• What level of maturity do you think is necessary before it is okay to start dating?

• What level of maturity do you think is necessary before becoming physically intimate?

• What personal development do you think needs to take place before you can be in a successful, fulfilling relationship?

• Do you think it's better to be friends first?

EXPLORING DATING AND BOUNDARIES

Think about what values are important to you in a dating relationship—and what rules will help uphold these—so that you can communicate these clearly to your child and have obvious guidelines in place.

• What dating activities are acceptable? How do these change as your child grows older?

• What qualities or attributes are valuable to you in a dating relationship?

• How much privacy do you think your child should be allowed to have when it comes to personal relationships?

• What boundaries do you think should be set for alone time together?

• How do you feel about co-ed group sleepovers? Are there boundaries that should be set for these?

• Is it ever okay for a child's boyfriend/ girlfriend to spend the night?

• How should physical boundaries be set? Such as, no private dates, no closed doors, etc.?

• What will you do if you discover that your child is being sexually intimate? How will your response differ depending on your child's age?

EXPLORING RELATIONSHIP IMPACT

Reflecting on the impact early relationships have, both in the present and in the future, will help you communicate to your child the value of making wise relationship decisions.

• What are your memories about your own first romantic relationship?

- How would you define "love"?

- How do you think your first relationship impacts future relationships?

- How do you think a romantic relationship impacts your quality of life as a teenager? What about as an adult?

- How do you think your own relationships impact your child's relationships?

- How much impact does your partner's personality have on your own personality? Is one of you more dominant than the other?

EXPLORING RELATIONSHIP INVOLVEMENT

It is a good idea to decide early on what level of involvement you think is appropriate for your child's relationships—this can be situational, depending on your child's personality, social circles, and level of maturity.

- Do you want to meet your child's significant other and her parents?

- What if you don't "approve" of your child's significant other? How will you manage this roadblock with your child?

- How involved do you think parents should be in their teen's early relationships?

- How involved do you think parents should be in later relationships?

- How prescriptive do you think family values should attempt to be?

- How do you plan to communicate these values to your child? Do you think it is important to do so before she is involved in a romantic relationship?

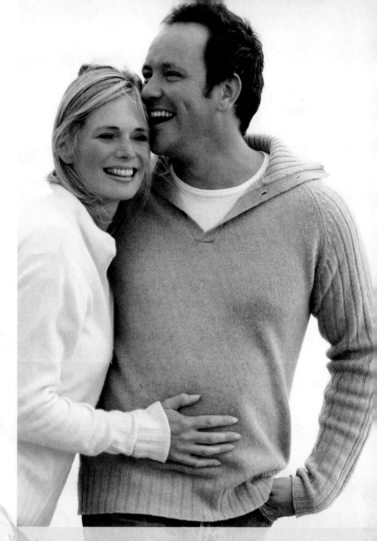

APPLYING YOUR ANSWERS Thinking about your relationship history can be painful or confusing. If you find that these questions are difficult to answer, it may be a good idea to talk about your feelings with a close friend or a therapist. Even if you have had harmful or damaged relationships in the past, you can pass along healthy values to your child and help guide early dating relationships. A good way to do this is to identify qualities in friendships or other relationships (respect, support, etc.) that are valuable to you, and then translate these to romantic relationships.

Your child's first relationship

Being involved in a romantic relationship can be one of the most rewarding parts of the human experience—this is why children seek to mimic adult relationships starting at such an early age. From the first crush to the first steady relationship, it is important to stay involved and interested in this important part of your child's life.

Crushes

Many children have crushes as early as 3 or 4 years old, perhaps developing an interest in another child in their preschool class or maybe a neighborhood playmate. During this time period, a crush is generally nothing more than children playing at adult roles. For example, your daughter might want to play house and pretend that her crush is her husband, or your son might call one of the girls in his class his "girlfriend." Children like to imitate adult behavior, and these crushes are harmless and generally based more on imagination than on reality. They are often forgotten within a few weeks' time. As your child grows, crushes will become more serious and will seem more real, but they will still be largely based on fantasy and romantic ideals.

The first steady relationship

There is a good chance that your child's first romantic relationship will happen sooner than you might anticipate, possibly as early as the end of elementary school or the start of junior high. As a parent, it is a good idea to decide with your partner what guidelines you want to set out for your child when it comes to these important milestones. For example, at what age do you think it is okay for her to have a steady boyfriend? At what age will you allow her to go on unsupervised dates? Setting guidelines ahead of time will not only help your child clearly understand what behavior is acceptable and what behavior is not acceptable, it will also help her to see that your rules are not arbitrary and created on a whim. If she has had plenty of time

>>> YOUR CHILD'S RELATIONSHIP IS MORE THAN JUST A CRUSH WHEN . . .

Crushes are a natural part of growing up. From preschool onward, your child will likely be interested both in friends at school and in celebrity figures. This is healthy and normal—and it is also healthy for this to move beyond a crush at a certain age, especially if you are able to maintain a degree of involvement in the relationship. Signs that your child is becoming more serious about someone include:
• Increasing need for privacy, especially when talking about a love interest
• Seeming angry or embarrassed when you ask questions about the person
• Acting moody and upset one day and giddy the next, or other behavior that signifies that her emotions are involved in the relationship

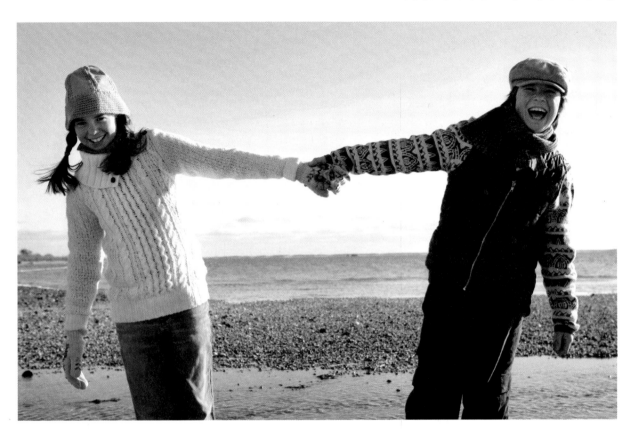

to process and digest your rules about dating, she will be more likely to understand that you and your partner have put time and thought into each restriction. Communicating and sticking to your rules will also help give your child a sense of guidance and support so she can make safe dating decisions that are in accordance with your family values and expectations. In addition, it will ensure that by the time your child becomes seriously interested in dating, you will have already established an ongoing conversation with her what it means to be in a healthy, fulfilling relationship.

One caveat: try to stay considerate of your child's needs as you set these guidelines, and beware of rules that are too strict and unbending. This is especially true when it comes to first dating experiences. Early relationships rarely last long or become serious, and if you allow your child small freedoms, you will help create an atmosphere of trust and respect as you each go through this turning point in the parent-child relationship.

Aim to make compromises that work for both of you. For example, if you don't believe that your child should be going out on individual dates with her first steady boyfriend, try inviting her boyfriend out for family dinners, or drop the couple off at the movie theater and pick them up afterward. Staying closely involved in their activities can help take some of the forbidden excitement out of the relationship, and redirect the focus to friendship and harmless flirting, while still allowing the relationship to develop. It will also give you a good chance to get to know the person your child is dating.

Dating

As a parent, you are able to play an important role in encouraging and celebrating healthy dating relationships. Just as you helped your child to form happy and healthy friendships, you should also be a guiding light when it comes to choosing a significant other, teaching about communication as a couple, and setting guidelines and boundaries for each stage of development.

Group dating

A good way to initiate your child into the dating world is to allow her to go on group dates. This gives a degree of autonomy, while also protecting against situations that might move too fast. Even in these group scenarios it is a good idea to find out details about your child's plans. A good rule of thumb, especially during the early teen years, is to ask that all group dating occurs in public places, such as the mall or movie theater. This will help ensure that the activities are healthy and fun, and that peer pressure of any kind is kept to a minimum.

It is also important to stay aware of who will be part of the group. If the group includes only friends that you have never met, spend some time talking with your child before she goes out. As teens get older, group dates do have the potential to become a breeding ground for peer pressure. In fact, group dates can sometimes be more intense than one-on-one dates, as teens can goad one another into pushing the envelope sexually. Even for a child with a strong sexual education and knowledge, this naturally competitive element can tempt her to take sexual steps that she otherwise would not.

In addition, even in group dating scenarios, it is important to make sure that your teenager only dates within her own age group, which means someone who is no more than 2 years older. Studies show that young women who date men outside of their age group are at higher risk for dangerous behaviors such as drinking, using drugs, and having sex. In fact, a study by the US National Center on Addiction and Substance Abuse at Columbia University found that 58 percent of girls who had boyfriends that were at least two years older drank alcohol, compared to just 25 percent of the girls who did not date or who dated boys within their age group. Similarly, 50 percent of girls who dated older boys smoked marijuana, compared to 8 percent of the other girls, and 65 percent of girls dating older boys smoked cigarettes, compared to 14 percent of girls who dated in their own age group. All of these activities can lead to earlier sexual activity—and indeed, further research reveals that two thirds of teenage moms in the United States were impregnated by men older than 20 years of age.

Monitoring dating relationships

One of the best ways to monitor your child's relationship is to get to know the person your child is dating. Taking an interest in his relationship will help your child feel more like an adult, and may also encourage him to open up more about the relationship. To minimize any embarrassment your child might feel, make this a fun invitation rather than an obligation.

Planning a dinner is a good way to ensure you can all talk and have concentrated time together, but if dinner is too threatening, try planning a more casual event, such as a day at an amusement park or at a concert in the park. **To extend the invitation, try saying**: "I have noticed that you and Alison are spending a lot of time together. I would love to get to know her since she is so important in your life."

It is also a good idea to monitor the balance in your child's life. Although the early stages of a relationship can be all-consuming, it is important to encourage your child to continue to value other friends, extracurricular activities, and school work. Remind your child that his friends deserve his energy and time as well, and that in order to have a happy and healthy relationship, he needs to be a well-rounded person with his own interests and personality. If this proves difficult, you may want to set some additional rules on time your child spends with his significant other, such as that they are only allowed to spend two nights a week hanging out.

Teaching by example

One of the best ways you can help your child choose healthy relationships is to practice what you preach. The example of a healthy marriage is the best gift that you can give to your child. If you and your partner are divorced, you can still encourage smart relationship decisions by continuing to treat your ex with respect.

If you are single and dating, think about how you might instruct your child through your own relationships. For example, if your family rule is that your teen waits until adulthood to have sex, you may not want to have your partner stay the night. Even though you are an adult, having someone spend the night can conflict with the values your child has been learning. Children often mimic their parents' behavior, especially when they already view themselves as adults.

WHAT TO SAY . . .
IF YOU THINK YOUR CHILD IS IN AN UNHEALTHY RELATIONSHIP

If you are concerned about your child's relationship for any reason find a private time when you can talk with your child. Stay open-minded and supportive, but share your concerns honestly.

CONVERSATION STARTER: Try saying, "You know I can't help but notice that you often seem upset after spending time with Jake or talking to him on the phone. Do you feel like this is true sometimes?"

Your child might become defensive after any negative comments about the relationship, no matter how well said. Minimize defensiveness by explaining more specifically what you've noticed and why you are concerned.

FOLLOW-UP: "Arguments are normal, but it seems like he might be not behaving as respectfully toward you as you deserve. Do you ever feel this way?"

Give your child plenty of time to process and respond to what you've said. Then make sure she knows you are available to listen, whether she wants to talk more now or in the future.

FOLLOW-UP: "I have had my fair share of disagreements with boyfriends in the past. If there is something you want to talk about, I am always here to listen, no matter what."

To end the conversation on a positive note, reiterate how important her happiness is to you and how you want her to always feel loved by the people she loves.

FOLLOW-UP: "I just want you to be happy and to have a boyfriend that makes you feel as special and priceless as you are. If [insert boyfriend's name] makes you feel this way, then I am glad. If not, I want to be sure you know that it's okay to have doubts and to think about whether this is really the relationship you want."

Monitoring time alone

Setting rules about how and when your child sees her significant other becomes especially important as she gets older. You can base these rules on your child's maturity and what you know about her relationship. A good goal is to maintain an atmosphere of trust that allows your child to make some decisions for herself, while keeping a level of involvement that protects against too much autonomy.

Setting rules

At each stage of your child's maturity, you will need to decide how to manage his privileges in the home. With a young teen—13 to 14 years old—setting the rule of no alone time with a significant other is feasible, especially if your family rule is that all dates must be group dates.

As your teen gets older and proves that he is mature enough to handle more responsibility, you may feel comfortable increasing his freedom by allowing him to go on individual dates and spend more time alone with his significant other. As he is allowed greater freedom, you can still restrict some of their alone time within your own home, such as by asking that they don't spend time in his bedroom with the door closed. Give your child some privacy, but also let him know that you will check in on him occasionally, so he knows that he will still be semi-supervised.

It is a good idea to ask about the restrictions in place in his significant other's home, as well. If her family isn't as involved or have different house rules, the temptation to spend time in the house with fewer restrictions will be great. Get to know his girlfriend and her family, and talk with her parents about your house rules. Make an effort even if the other parents seem unwilling or uninterested, and remind them that you would like your rules to be followed as much as possible. If you are truly uncomfortable with the lack of supervision they provide, you can ask your child that he and his girlfriend spend time at your house instead. If this is the case, try to make her feel as welcome as possible. A child who doesn't have involved parents craves this type of parental support and encouragement, so your involvement will feel like a gift to her, rather than a punishment.

Spending the night together

Most parents are not comfortable with their child spending the night alone with their significant other, and this is understandable. Allowing teens to spend the night alone together is very risky. One in five kids have sex before the age of 15, and only 30 percent of parents know about it—even though the intimacy is likely occurring under their own roof! Be especially vigilant around coed sleepovers and parties such as prom night, or some other activity where alcohol is likely to be involved. It is a good idea to set a rule that your child cannot spend the night alone with his girlfriend, even if you are in the house with him. You can keep this rule even with college-aged children that are returning to the house for the summer or for an extended vacation. In your own home at least, family rules about coed sleepovers don't have to change as your child gets older.

TEACHABLE MOMENTS
TALKING TO YOUR TEEN ABOUT ALONE TIME

It can be difficult to decide how to manage when your teen can be alone with a significant other. Start this conversation early, and stress to your child that alone time is a privilege, not a right, and that it can be taken away if you feel behavior is inappropriate.

• **AFTER WATCHING A MOVIE:** After watching a movie that shows teens abusing alone time, such as by trashing the house or by having sex at a young age, start a conversation with your child about what you've seen. You might say something like: "You know in that movie last night the main character really abused his parents' trust. I want you to have privacy and enjoy time alone with your girlfriend, but not if you are doing things that are against our family rules." Explain that if your child respects your boundaries about alone time, you will promise to respect his privacy in return.

• **AFTER OVERHEARING A CONVERSATION:** If you overhear your child and his friends talking about sex or any type of physical intimacy, you can use this as a conversation bridge. Later, when you are alone and you have time to talk privately, say something like "I was a bit concerned when I heard you and your friends talking about relationships the other day. While I think it is fine to date and I trust you and your friends, I want you to understand that I don't think relationships should be physically intimate until you are older." If your child is in a relationship, let him know that he can come to you with questions or concerns about intimacy at any time.

• **AT THE START OF A NEW RELATIONSHIP:** When your child is in the early stages of a relationship, use this opportunity to remind her of your house rules, especially as they may change as she grows older. You might say: "I am so excited to hear about Bobby. He sounds like a really nice guy, and I can't wait to meet him. Just remember that it is fine for him to spend time here, but if you're hanging out in your bedroom, the door must be open."

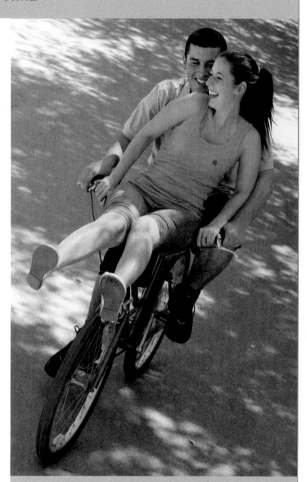

CONVERSATION STARTER 1: "You have made some good decisions lately, and as a result, we think that you and [insert significant other's name] are ready to be at home when we're not here. Just remember the other talks we've had about maintaining boundaries."

CONVERSATION STARTER 2: "I know some of your other friends have their boyfriends spend the night, but as we've talked about, we don't think this is a good idea for you. Do you understand why?"

Setting physical boundaries

Helping your child set physical boundaries for his relationship can be a difficult conversation to initiate—but it can also be a very important step in helping him develop a sense of sexual responsibility. Remember that the sooner you start stressing the importance of sexual values, the more likely these lessons will become part of your child's decisions about physical boundaries.

Emotional intimacy

Start by having a discussion about the different levels of intimacy, including emotional intimacy. It can be easy to forget that physical attraction is just one part of the equation. For many teenagers, their first romantic relationship does not just entail a first date or first kiss, but also the first time they talk and share private parts of themselves with someone outside of their close family. This is particularly true for teenage boys. While girls tend to be more open and talkative with their friends, boys often bottle up their feelings and private thoughts. A teenage boy's first romantic relationship might be the first time he opens up and starts releasing some of those long-hidden feelings, which explains why first relationships can feel so heady and powerful, even without the physical connection.

Physical intimacy

Outline the levels of physical intimacy, or "bases," as shown on pages 128-129. Once you have defined these levels, it is a good idea to discuss the fact that sexual intimacy can quickly escalate and jump further ahead before either partner is truly ready. Give particular attention to oral and manual sex. Many teens don't view oral sex as sex, so it is important to stress the fact that it is just as dangerous from a health

perspective as intercourse, and that it is just as emotionally destructive if engaged in too soon. Additionally, other forms of sex, such as manual sex, can lead teens to a point where they physically don't want to stop, even though they are emotionally unprepared for this step.

Talking about intimacy with a partner

As part of the conversation about intimacy, it is important to directly address how to broach this topic in a relationship. If you equip your teen with the ability to say no to sexual advances that go against your family values and give her tips for setting boundaries while on dates or in a relationship, you are taking a big step in promoting smart relationship decisions.

The first step is encouraging your teen not to get caught up in being "nice" or "polite." Young women especially are often raised to be people-pleasers, and saying no to someone (even if it is about something that they feel is wrong) can make them feel guilty. Let your daughter know that saying no isn't just a gift for herself—it's a gift for her date as well. If she isn't ready to have sex, then having sex isn't fair to her or her partner. The same is true for teenage boys. Unless both partners feel prepared and comfortable, the emotional fallout of rushing into sex might be more overwhelming and damaging than either partner realizes.

It is equally important to prepare your teen for the different arguments she might encounter if she refuses sex. Her boyfriend might say: "But I love you" or "If you loved me, you would do this for me," or "We are going to be together forever, anyway, so why do we have to wait?" or "If you won't have sex with me, then some other girl will." Explain to your teen that real love respects boundaries and never tries to push someone into sex—and that if she and her significant other are going to be together forever, then they have their whole lives ahead of them to have sex. Let your child know that any time someone tries to push her into having sex it is disrespectful and manipulative, and not how a healthy relationship functions. As part of this conversation, teach your teen that any decisions to take a step toward greater intimacy should be discussed beforehand in a calm, non-sexually charged atmosphere.

Talking with teenage boys

Teenage boys should hear the same lessons about setting and respecting boundaries, although they may be less likely to feel as pressured to have sex. Encourage your son to be respectful of his partner's body, and tell him that he should never try to convince someone to have sex when she says "no." Oftentimes, boys believe that no is simply a girl's way of playing hard to get. Inform your son that this is not the case, and that he should always respect someone's decision not to have sex.

You can also help your son understand the emotional expectations that may come along with sex. For example, does he know that he wants to stay with this person? Does he understand that she will have more expectations of him afterward, and that she will expect them to stay together? Guiding your child through these possible outcomes can help him think of sex as a responsibility and not just a temptation.

WHAT TO SAY . . .
IF YOU THINK YOUR CHILD IS CROSSING PHYSICAL BOUNDARIES

If you discover that your child is crossing physical boundaries or engaging in sexual behavior that you find inappropriate, find a private time to have a conversation. Try to stay approachable and open, so that you have a real discussion and not just a lecture.

CONVERSATION STARTER: "I am a little concerned about something and I want to talk to you about it. I really want us to have an honest, open relationship because I think that you deserve to have my support and unconditional love at all times."

You can pause to give your child a chance to respond before beginning to directly discuss your concerns about the relationship.

FOLLOW-UP: "You are usually very honest with me in return, which is why I am surprised that you haven't talked to me about your decision to take things to the next level with Anna."

Pause again to give your child a chance to open up about the decisions he has made and how he is feeling about his relationship.

FOLLOW-UP: "I know that we have talked about the importance of waiting. I also know that it is ultimately your decision how to handle the physical side of your relationship, but I just want to say again how much I hope you and your girlfriend don't rush into something you might later regret."

Encourage your child to reflect and possibly share further by asking direct questions about his own thoughts and sexual values.

FOLLOW UP: "Have you thought about any of this or talked about this with your girlfriend? What physical boundaries do you feel are important for your relationship at this stage, if any? How have these changed since you first started dating, and why?"

LEARNING ABOUT LEVELS OF PHYSICAL INTIMACY

From sharing that first kiss to having sex for the first time, negotiating the stages of physical intimacy can be fraught with complication and confusion. When your child starts to think about dating, around the age of 12–13, talk to him about affection, sexual desires, and feelings to help him understand and make the right choices about physical intimacy. There are four main levels of intimacy, which are often described using well-known baseball terms.

AFTER THIS LESSON YOUR CHILD WILL BE MORE LIKELY TO...

- Understand what each stage of intimacy involves on a physical level
- Appreciate that each level of physical intimacy requires deeper emotional involvement and maturity
- Realize that physical intimacy can lead to a bruised ego, disappointment, and hurt if he goes too far, too soon
- Understand that third and fourth bases are not to be undertaken lightly
- Feel comfortable about saying "no" to physical intimacy—even if he is under pressure
- Realize that by having sex for the wrong reasons, there can be long-term physical and emotional consequences.

1 WHY DO WE CALL THEM BASES?

The concept of the "bases" is one that arose out of America's favorite pastime, baseball. The idea was that a couple would choose to touch certain bases—historically, first base was kissing, second base was touching breasts, third base was touching genitals, and a home run was, of course, intercourse. Today, the bases have become easy to pass, and have also changed in definition. The average teen now considers second base to be touching everything, third base to be oral sex, sometimes even anal sex, and a home run to be intercourse or, in some cases, multiple partners at once! To make sure you're on the same page, it's important to talk to your teen about these levels. Ask how he defines each base. What are his peers doing? What bases are considered normal for his age group and what, if anything, is considered to be going too far? You can then share your definition of the bases, stressing the importance of reflecting carefully and communicating openly before you decide to move on to each new stage of intimacy.

2 WHAT HAPPENS AT FIRST BASE?

First base is the starting point for physical intimacy. It is all about kissing, cuddling, and affection. It's the stage when a boy and girl are getting to know each other, going on first dates, holding hands, and gazing into each other's eyes. Is it okay to kiss someone on a first date? What does your child think? Explain that it can have less to do with timing and more to do with feelings. Do you like this person? Do you think she likes you back? Do you feel comfortable with this person? Do you trust her and her intentions toward you? Are you willing to risk your feelings on a kiss with somebody you do not know well or trust yet? These are the sorts of things you need to consider when thinking about whether or not to kiss someone.

3 WHAT'S SECOND BASE ALL ABOUT?

Second base means petting and deep kissing. Usually, it describes light petting above the waist so a boy might touch a girl's breasts, for example. You could explain that it's natural for teens to be curious about each other's bodies and want to explore what physical closeness feels like. Say that these sexual feelings are very exciting and sometimes quite difficult to control. Ask your teen how he would feel if his partner wanted to go further. Stress that your child should never go further than he wants to, or make decisions that he feels conflict with your family values. Kissing and petting with someone is not a promise of something more later, so he is not leading someone on or being a tease because he wants to stop. These actions should be part of a relationship built on trust, caring, respect, and friendship, so anyone who tries to make him feel bad about wanting to stop is not worthy of his affection in the first place.

4 TO GO TO THIRD BASE OR NOT?

Third base is generally considered to involve heavy petting, or touching and caressing each other's genitals. At what stage of a relationship does your child think it would be appropriate to get to this base? Does it depend on how long he has been dating? Should he be in love? This is a good point to bring up your family values again. Explain to your teen that this level of physical intimacy requires a great deal of mutual trust, respect, and understanding between two people. Because he is sharing more of his body and his heart, he has to be very careful to protect against being hurt emotionally. Many teens view oral sex as a third-base activity because it doesn't involve intercourse. You might want to point out to your child that oral sex is every bit as intimate as intercourse and should never be entered into lightly. Neither is it a safe alternative to sex—you might not get pregnant but you can get an STD during oral sex just as easily as you can during intercourse.

5 WHEN IS IT TIME FOR FOURTH BASE?

Fourth base is the stage at which full sexual intercourse takes place. You might want to point out here that while baseball is a competitive sport, intimacy and sex are anything but. Lots of teenagers do have a competitive mentality about getting to fourth base first—boys in particular may try to "score" in this way. Let your child know that he should never coerce anyone or feel coerced into doing anything he feels uncomfortable with at any time. You can also ask the "big" questions during this talk. When does your child think the right time to have sex might be? Why does he think that there's a legal age of consent? Now's the time to talk about the emotional and physical consequences of sex and the importance of being mature enough to cope. By having sex before he is ready, your child is opening himself up to feelings like guilt, shame, and regret. Focus on helping your teen think about what makes a relationship strong. Talk about what it means to truly care for another person and what sex should be like—as part of a mature, loving, respectful relationship.

HOW TO ANSWER QUESTIONS ABOUT LEVELS OF PHYSICAL INTIMACY

Your child is likely to have lots of questions about physical intimacy and sexual behavior. Being able to communicate openly, honestly, and without embarrassment about these issues is essential in order for your child to feel comfortable approaching you for advice and information.

Q. What does "petting" mean?
A. Petting means intimate touching and can happen either with clothes or without. Sometimes it can be lighter (such as a boy touching a girl's breast over her clothing) and sometimes it can be very intimate (as with manual sex).

Q. Is oral sex really sex?
A. It is definitely sexual behavior. Some people consider it as even more intimate than intercourse; others see it as being less personal. You have to decide for yourself what values you place on different types of sexual behavior.

Learning together

First love

Falling in love is a priceless experience—and also a challenging one. Stay involved in your child's first true romance by supporting the relationship, sharing your own love history, and instructing on the difference between love and lust. Making yourself an available resource for questions and concerns will help keep you involved and influential during this important milestone.

The impact of first love

Your first love can be the model on which you fashion every future relationship. If your first boyfriend was respectful and faithful, you will likely leave the relationship with a healthy self-confidence and a good opinion of men and dating. If your first boyfriend cheated on you or pressured you to have sex before you were ready, you might suffer from a lifetime of low self-esteem or a lack of sexual enjoyment. Indeed, many people who had a negative sexual initiation suffer decades later from a damaged sexual outlook and feelings of shame and regret.

As you prepare your child for this experience, it is a good idea to talk about the difference between lust and love. Many teens (and even some adults) misinterpret these first feelings of attraction for something deeper. Talking about how desire can sometimes cloud one's decision-making process can help encourage your child to more closely process and label her emotions.

Supporting your child's relationship

In order to stay involved in your child's relationship, it is important to offer respectful support from the beginning. Parents often wrongly think that if they take their teenager's relationship seriously, it will encourage him to take the relationship to the next level of intimacy. Instead, respecting your child's relationship is about demonstrating that you value his relationship because it is important to him. Supporting your child and validating his feelings won't make him any more likely to make adult decisions—but it will make him more likely to come to you for advice and listen to your opinions on sex and love.

Supporting early relationships includes avoiding patronizing comments. Not only will these hurt your child's feelings, they may also drive a wedge into your communication—which is the last thing you want to do when he is making his first forays into the world of sex and love. If it is difficult for you to view your child's relationship as a serious commitment, try to remember how it felt to be in that early flush of love. Remembering—and possibly sharing about—your own early relationships will help you relate to your teenager on a level that will encourage him to be emotionally vulnerable.

For example, the next time your child seems upset or moody after talking to his girlfriend on the phone, say something like, "I notice that you seemed sad after talking to Laura. That reminds me of a time that I got in a fight with my first girlfriend. I was upset for four days—I will never forget it." Your child may want to know more about your story, and as you share these details, he may feel more comfortable opening up to you about his own relationship.

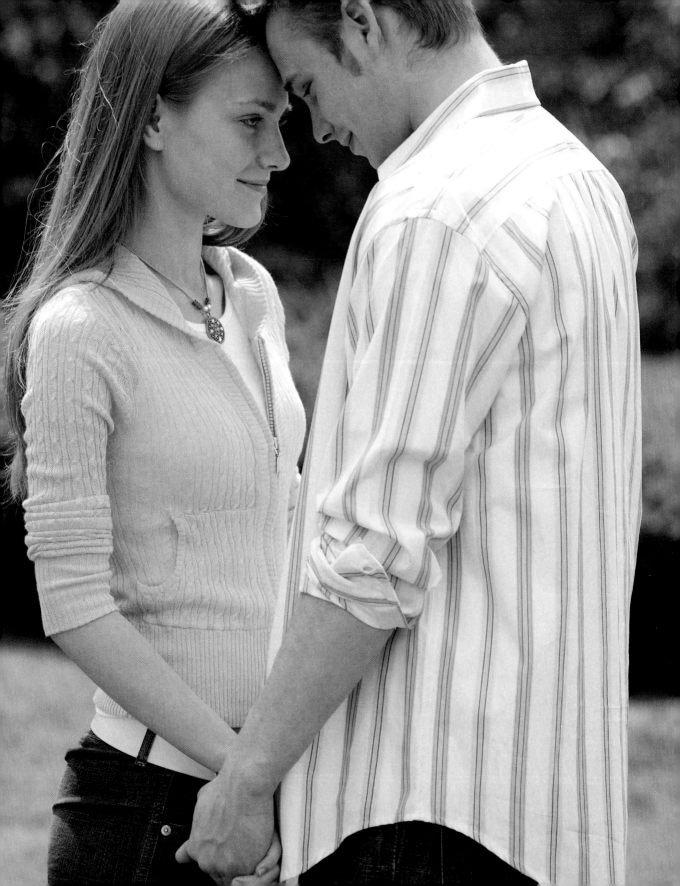

Dealing with heartbreak

Inevitably, your child's first breakup will be difficult, but it can also provide an opportunity to learn important life lessons. Aim to use this time to teach your child about the realities and risks of love, and about how to heal from difficult experiences. Staying active and looking to become involved in new activities are good ways to emerge from heartbreak as a stronger person.

Showing empathy

The first breakup can be a very painful part of childhood. As a parent, it can sometimes be difficult to know how to relate to your child during this time, especially if the relationship has been short. Keep in mind that while six months may seem brief, that same period represents one-thirtieth of a 15-year-old's life!

One of the best ways to empathize with your child is simply to spend time together. Whether your teenager is into theater, sports, or art, plan a day that focuses on her interests. Offering support and giving her control over the day—even if she simply wants to do nothing—is a good way to nurture her during this time.

You can also take this opportunity to explain the realities of love. Your child's first breakup might be the only time she has been confronted with the reality of what happens when love doesn't work out. Talk with your teen about the risk involved whenever you love someone. A good way to do this is by sharing about your own first breakup and how you felt afterward.

Encouraging proactive healing

In addition to offering verbal and moral support, it is a good idea to encourage your child to be proactive in the healing process. This can help your child's life return to normal more quickly.

The good news about teen breakups is that they often do have a capacity to heal at a fast pace, provided there are other parts of life that keep your child busy and involved.

One simple way to promote this is to help your child stick to her routine. Many parents make the mistake of allowing their teenager complete freedom after a breakup. One day off school post-breakup might be helpful in giving your teen time to cry it out, but giving additional time off will only prolong the grief process. Sticking to a routine of school and normal activities will keep her mind occupied on the present rather than the past. Practicing regular chores and responsibilities can also help provide a sense of normalcy and even accomplishment.

You can also help your child by getting her engaged in community activities, such as visiting the elderly at a nursing home or volunteering at a local animal shelter. One of the main reasons teenage breakups can be so painful is because teens have a hard time thinking outside of their own needs and feelings. This can complicate the healing process, since your child might not have a clear frame of reference for how she is feeling. In other words, she might not realize that her relationship isn't the only thing in her life worth thinking about. Volunteering can help her realize that there are other people in the world that are hurting as well, and can give her a boost of happiness and self-esteem.

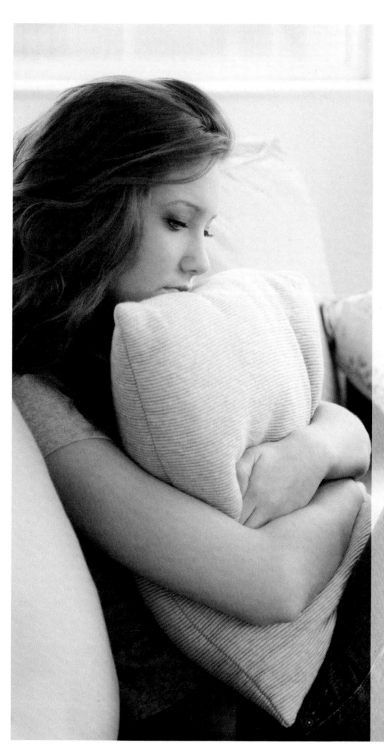

WHAT TO SAY . . .
AFTER A BREAKUP

....

During this time, your teen might not be very open to talking about what happened, and she might even resent you or try to blame you for the breakup, especially if she feels like your rules were too restrictive. Try to ignore any misplaced anger and instead stick to the issue at hand—her sadness over the breakup. While it might seem like there is nothing you can say to help her feel better, remember that she is still a child and relies on you for comfort and support.

Conversation starter: "I am sorry about your relationship with Chris. I know you guys were very close and that you weren't expecting to breakup so suddenly."

Wait for a while to see your child's response. This conversation should be more about listening than about saying the right words.

Follow up: "I wish I could say something to make it all go away, but since I can't, I just want you to know that I am here to listen to you whenever you want. Is there any part of your relationship that you want to talk about? Do you have any questions about what happened?"

Your child may open up at this point, or she may remain silent. The important thing is that she knows that you are there to support her.

Follow up: "I don't always have all the right answers, but I love you very much and I want to be here for you during this hard time. Please know that if you ever want to share about this or talk about your feelings, you can always come to me."

Encouraging healthy relationships

As your child grows into adulthood, you will eventually need to allow her to make her own decisions regarding sex, love, and romance. Teaching early lessons about what it means to be in a healthy relationship is the best way to protect her future happiness. In addition, learning to support and accept her will help ensure your relationship is happy, loving, and honest.

What is a healthy relationship?

Healthy relationships are relationships that are age-appropriate, meaning that the couple doesn't engage in sexual behavior until both parties are emotionally mature enough to make this decision. They are relationships in which both partners continue to have their own lives, their own friendships, and their own goals. Healthy relationships are ones that complement your child's life, rather than take away from it, and build her up, rather than tear her down.

Forming a healthy relationship isn't easy, for teenagers or for adults. If your teenager witnessed an unhealthy relationship in progress as she grew up, she might have adopted certain unhealthy behaviors as her own, even if only subconsciously. Maybe she never learned how to communicate her feelings, or how to get into an argument without yelling. No one's childhood is perfect, and you shouldn't feel guilty if you think your child might have developed some unhealthy relationship behavior. Instead, you might consider getting therapy as a family, or individual therapy just for your child. Having an unbiased person to talk to can be very helpful for your teen during this time.

Part of encouraging healthy relationships means exhibiting healthy relationships in your life. If you are respectful of your partner, confident and independent, your child will have a better chance of growing up to be respectful of his partners and to be confident and independent. If you exhibit unhealthy behavior, such as yelling, cheating, lying, or manipulation, your child will learn to behave that way within his romantic relationships as well.

Dealing with inappropriate flirting

If you think that your child may be developing an unhealthy relationship or behaving inappropriately, don't ignore it. For example, if your teenager is dating or flirting with someone much older, talk to her about what you see happening. Perhaps she is acting out for attention from her peers, or maybe she is attracted to the idea of dating someone so much older and experienced.

Rather than becoming angry and yelling at her, say something like, "I am worried that you are talking to someone who is five years older than you. I know you say that you are just flirting and joking around, but I think we need to discuss why you want to talk to someone who is much older. What about the situation do you find so appealing? Have the two of you talked about the age difference at all?"

If your child won't talk to you about how she is feeling, consider taking her to someone she may be able to open up to, such as a therapist, a close family friend, or a religious advisor.

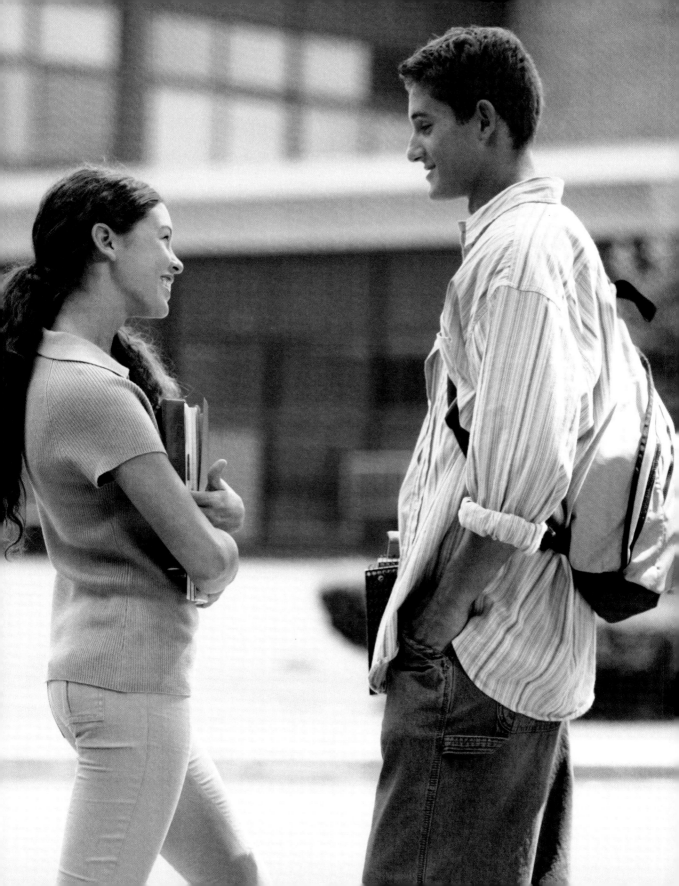

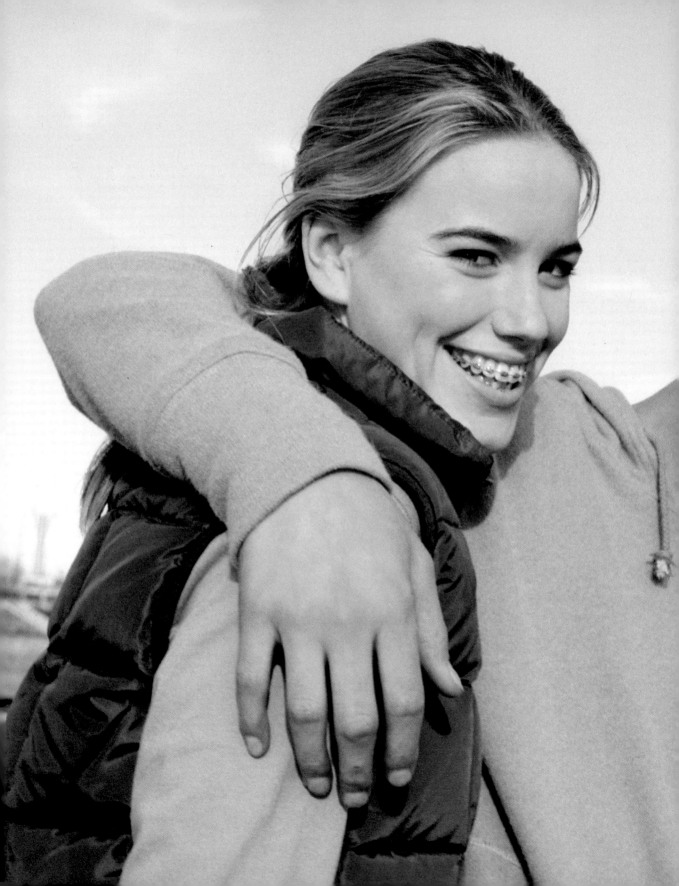

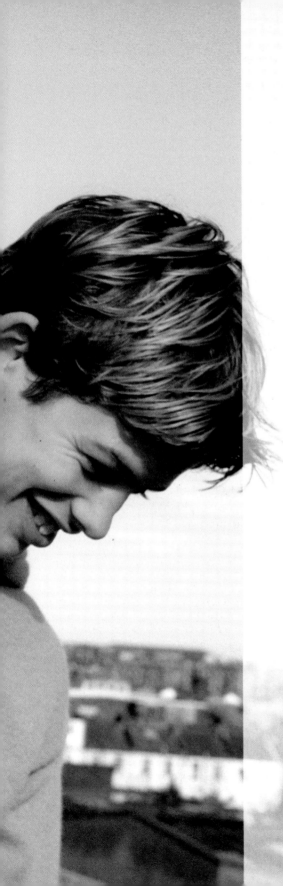

6

TALKING ABOUT SEXUAL RELATIONSHIPS

ASSESSING YOUR VALUES: SEXUAL RELATIONSHIPS

Sexual relationships are a reality for millions of teenagers. Whether or not your teenager engages in sex is ultimately not up to you—however, you can decide when and how you want to supply him with knowledge about staying emotionally and physically safe. Consider the following questions to help clarify your feelings and beliefs about teenage sexual activity, then discuss these feelings with your partner.

EXPLORING SEXUAL INTIMACY

Think about the qualities that are important for deep intimacy, so you can teach your child to value these as she begins to make her own sexual decisions.

• What qualities do you think should be present in a relationship before any level of true sexual intimacy occurs (e.g. manual sex, oral sex, etc.)?

• How do you think sex contributes to intimacy in a relationship, and vice versa?

• Would you be able to accept your child's decision to become sexually intimate, even if you didn't agree with it?

• Do you have any negative feelings regarding your own sexual history, or the age you chose to become intimate for the first time?

• Do you think men and women think about and experience intimacy differently?

• What non-sexual acts do you think can create and build intimacy?

EXPLORING SEXUAL RISK

Sexual risks can be both physical and emotional. Reflect on what things you want to protect your child from, so that you can better communicate these concerns.

• What are the emotional risks that come with a sexual relationship? How do these differ from the risks in a non-sexual relationship?

• What are the physical risks?

• What are your major fears concerning your child's sex life (e.g. heartbreak, pregnancy, etc.)?

• What risk do you think is involved with sexual acts such as oral or anal sex? How do these differ from the risks of intercourse?

• What outside factors do you think can increase sexual risks (e.g. alcohol, drugs, etc.)?

EXPLORING SEXUAL PROTECTION

Think in advance about how you want to communicate information on this important topic, so that your child has the knowledge and awareness to make smart decisions that are informed by your family's values.

• What information do you want your child to know about contraception?

• How much do you value abstinence? Do you think this is a realistic goal for teens?

• What is your motivation for encouraging your child to stay abstinent (e.g. religious or moral beliefs, health concerns, etc.)?

- What guidelines will you try to set regarding your child's sexual activity (e.g. don't have sex until you are married, until you are out of the house, until you are an adult, etc.)?

- Do you support giving condoms and/or contraceptives to teenagers? How do you feel about telling your child where he can find these if he decides to have sex (e.g. family planning clinic, doctor's office, etc.)?

- Do you think it is important to talk to your child about safer sex practices as they apply to other forms of intercourse, such as oral sex and anal sex? Why or why not?

- How important do you think it is to talk about and plan for sexual protection with a partner before you make the decision to have sex?

EXPLORING SEXUAL DECISIONS

Teaching your child to make careful, well-thought-out sexual decisions is one of the best tools you can give her.

- How much were you impacted by peer pressure as a child? Did it ever lead you to take sexual steps that you later regretted?

- What do you think are valid reasons to enter into a sexual relationship? How can you encourage your child to reflect on this?

- Have you ever set sexual goals for yourself or your relationship? Do you think it would be beneficial for your child to do this?

- How open do you want your conversations with your child to be when it comes to sexual decisions? Would you want her to come to you with questions or concerns, or would you rather she talk to someone else, such as a trusted family friend or an older sibling?

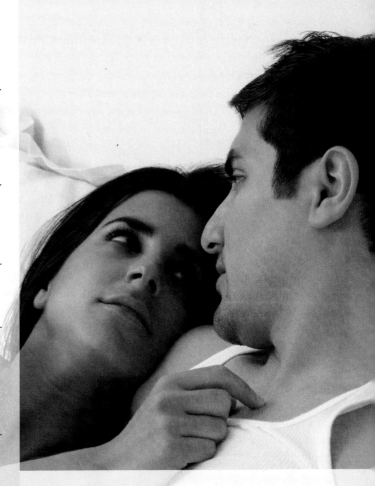

APPLYING YOUR ANSWERS These questions can be difficult to answer, because they force you to stop thinking of your son or daughter as a child, and to acknowledge that sexual desires and risks will become an increasingly important part of life during the journey to adulthood. However, making these decisions is a crucial part of protecting your child from possible pain, both emotional and physical. Take plenty of time to establish values that you both feel comfortable with, and that you feel can protect and guide your child throughout adolescence and adulthood.

Your child's intimate relationship

Relationships differ from adolescence to adulthood—which you probably know already, having gone through both yourself. However, adolescent relationships should still be treated with respect, particularly as intimacy increases. A supportive attitude will encourage your child to be more open, which in turn will give you opportunities to offer guidance on sexual decision-making.

The first intimate relationship

Most parents will experience their child going through a variety of crushes and casual relationships, so it can be difficult to know when he has actually moved on to a more serious relationship—and everything that might entail, including physical and emotional intimacy. The best barometer you have to judge your child's relationship is conversation. Talk to him about his relationship, and try to ask questions that will illuminate the seriousness of the relationship. Your child might be hesitant or shy to speak at first, but the more you seem genuinely interested in his relationship—as opposed to anxious or judgmental—the more he will feel safe sharing these personal details.

For example, you might ask: "How long have you and Kate been together now? Almost a year, right? That's a long time. Do you ever talk about the future? Do you think you will try to apply to the same colleges? If you go to different schools, will you try to maintain a long-distance relationship, or do you think you will break up?"

Communication in teenage relationships

The biggest difference between teenage relationships and adult relationships is the teenager's ability to communicate effectively. Unlike adults who have had time to discover how to communicate with others in general, and with their significant other in particular, teenagers are just beginning to learn these

>>> **YOUR CHILD'S RELATIONSHIP IS BECOMING MORE INTIMATE IF...**

Talking openly with your teen about her relationship is one of the best ways to stay in touch with the stage of your child's relationship—and also with the likelihood of physical intimacy. Other signs that your child is progressing to a sexual relationship (or is already involved in a sexual relationship) may include:

• Desiring more privacy and space, particularly in her bedroom (which might be where she keeps birth control or other items she may not want you to find)

• Asking for more freedom with her curfew and nightly activities

• Experiencing mood swings that she can't fully explain, especially if these relate to time spent with her significant other

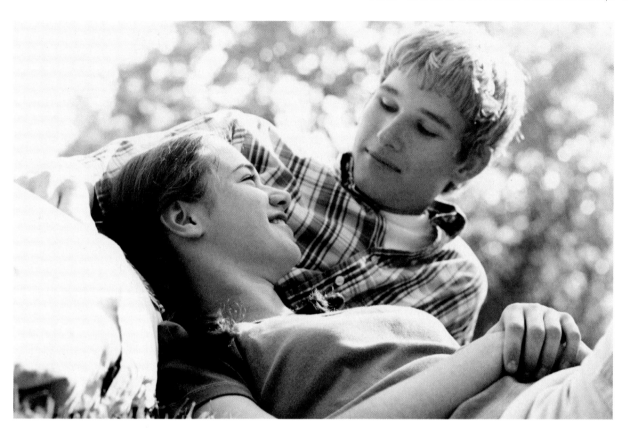

lessons, particularly when it comes to dating relationships. For example, a teenage girl might feel angry with her boyfriend but pretend like nothing is wrong until weeks later when she finally breaks down, or a teenage boy might not be able to express "I love you" to his girlfriend even though he wants to.

The combination of poor communication and budding hormones means that teenage relationships tend to be short-lived but quite intense—which is why your teenager might become very upset after ending a relationship that lasted only a few months. Power struggles often play a big role in teenage relationship dynamics, and you may notice this in your child's early relationships as she begins to discover what it means to be in love. You may also notice that negative feedback from peers will deter your child from a relationship—while alternately, enough parental disapproval can serve to cement the relationship. This is all part of the teenage experience of seeking autonomy and struggling to define personal identity.

As your teen continues to date and learn from experience, her ability to communicate and express her feelings will improve, and her relationships will deepen and grow as a result. You will notice her beginning to feel more comfortable and confident in her worth as a relationship partner, and also beginning to place more value and priority on her partner's feelings and needs. All of this will help your child develop greater maturity and a healthier self-esteem, which means fewer fights and breakups, and more healthy, serious, developed, and adult-like relationships.

Sex and intimacy

It is a good idea to start having conversations about the emotional connection that comes along with sex as you talk about physical information and concerns. Helping your child understand the deeper meaning of sex can go a long way in postponing intimacy. You can also introduce your child to other paths to intimacy that will progress a relationship, but that aren't purely physical.

Sex and emotions

Often when parents discuss sex with their children, they tend to focus on the physical risks, such as pregnancy or STDs, or their religious or moral reasons for abstinence. Remember that it's also good to talk about the link between sexual activity and emotions.

A good way to start this conversation is to talk to your teen about how sex in real life isn't like it is in the movies, with romantic music and candlelight. Nor is it always mutually pleasurable. While you shouldn't scare your teen from ever wanting to have sex, you can explain that real sex can be awkward, especially the first time, and that this is why you should wait until you are with someone you trust and feel safe sharing your body and soul with.

For example, you might say: "Have you noticed how sex seems so easy in the movies? In real life, sex can be romantic, but it isn't always perfect. You don't just bare your body when you have sex; you also bare your soul."

As part of this conversation, you can also talk to your teenager about how to increase intimacy in her relationship without sexual activity. Teenagers tend to see relationships as linear and growing toward sexual activity. However, there are many different ways to be emotionally intimate with a partner, some of which do not include intercourse. Try to give your teen some ideas of ways she can increase intimacy in her relationship without having sex, such as by introducing him to the family. By creating a bond that isn't purely physical, your teen can build a healthy foundation for a time when she does decide to have sex.

Male and female perspectives

When men and women reach orgasm, their brains are flooded with oxytocin, otherwise known as the "cuddle" hormone. Oxytocin creates feel-good emotions and feelings of bonding. Research suggests that male levels of testosterone counteract this release of oxytocin, minimizing its effect. In other words, while women are experiencing an oxytocin "high," men might not feel the same intimacy.

Thus, while a teenage girl might feel very bonded with her partner after sex, a teenage boy might feel unattached. Of course, this isn't true in every situation. However, it's important to talk to your teenagers about how these hormones might affect their sexual experience. **Try saying something like:** "I know I have taught you that boys and girls are equal, and they are. But that doesn't mean that we are the same. Men and women have different hormones that affect the way they think and feel, and some of your hormones might make you feel in love with your partner after you have sex."

TEACHABLE MOMENTS
TALKING ABOUT INTIMACY

Finding everyday moments to discuss intimacy with your child can make these very personal conversations feel more natural, and will also encourage your child to feel more comfortable coming to you with questions or concerns.

• **IN THE SUPERMARKET:** After reading the headlines about a teenage celebrity couple breaking up, talk with your teen about how much more difficult break-ups can be if sexual intimacy is involved. For example, "Did you hear about [insert star couple's name] breaking up? [Celebrity name] seemed pretty upset about it in the story I read. After you have sex with someone, that level of intimacy can make breaking up even more difficult, especially if the breakup is shortly after you have sex."

• **DURING A BREAKUP:** Use this time to talk to your teen about how he is feeling, and about how much more complicated those feelings can be after sexual intimacy. For example, "I was sorry to hear that you decided to break up with Tori, she was a nice girl. Was she very upset, or did she understand that you didn't want to get too serious with anyone right now? You know, once you have sex, breaking up becomes even harder, especially for girls. That's why it's really not a good idea to have casual sex with someone, or to have sex with them before you are ready to take things to the next level."

• **WHILE TALKING ABOUT SAFER SEX:** Safer sex isn't just about being safe physically, so take this opportunity to branch into a conversation about how to be safe emotionally as well. For example, say, "I know that you know how to protect yourself from STDs and pregnancy, but sex can also be risky because it involves your emotions. When you have sex with someone, you let them into your body and your soul. This intimacy can be very intense, and should only be shared between two people who love each other and trust each other 100%."

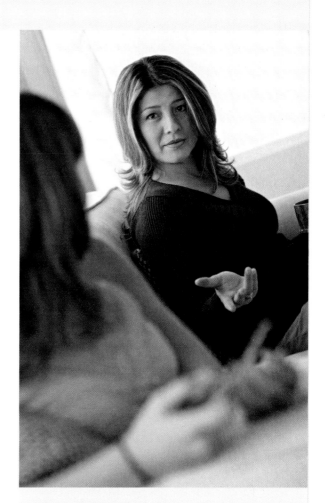

CONVERSATION STARTER 1: "It can be so hard to stay together, especially when you are exploring first relationships. That's why it is a good idea to wait to have sex, so that you don't commit more physically than you are ready to commit emotionally."

CONVERSATION STARTER 2: "What do you think about this celebrity couple's statement that they aren't sleeping together? I think that is a very wise and mature decision."

Teaching about sexual risk

There is a lot of information to cover when talking about sexual risk. Start an ongoing conversation about these risks, in order to give your child as much information as possible about STDs and teenage pregnancy. Knowledge truly is power, and the more your child knows about the risks that come along with sexual activity, the more equipped he will be to make smart sexual decisions.

Types of STDs

When your child begins puberty, it is time to start talking about safer sex, and about how sexual activity of all kinds, including oral sex, anal sex, and intercourse, can lead to STDs. It is a good idea to talk specifically about how young people have some of the highest STD rates in the country. Make sure to emphasize the fact that anyone can have a STD, and that symptoms are rarely apparent to the naked eye. Regular STD testing and practicing safer sex every single time is the only way to prevent STD infections—and even then, abstinence is the only true protection against sexual disease.

Next, review the common types of STD and their symptoms and treatments.

HPV: HPV is the most prevalent STD in the United States. Many people don't realize they have HPV, as the virus generally does not have any symptoms, although it can sometimes be indicated by warts around the genitals or anus. The Center for Disease Control and Prevention estimates that nearly 50% of sexually active individuals have HPV. Moreover, even if safe sex is practiced, the virus can still be spread. Recent studies have linked HPV to cervical cancer, genital warts, and precancerous lesions. This is especially scary for young women, since even benign cervical cancer can lead to infertility.

Although there is no cure for HPV, there is now a vaccine that can help protect young women between the ages of 9-26 against two forms of the virus. It can also help individuals who have already been infected with HPV from contracting other strains of the virus. This vaccine is most effective when given before a person becomes sexually active, so it is especially recommended for young girls. You don't have to tell your child details about the vaccine—simply say that it will prevent her from getting cervical cancer later in life. A vaccine for boys is also being researched.

Chlamydia: Increasing rates of chlamydia over the past few years have made it the second most widespread STD in the United States. Teenagers have an increased risk of contracting this disease—young women and men under 25 have the highest rates of chlamydia in the United States. Chlamydia is easily transmitted if safer sex is not practiced; however, condoms can decrease one's risk.

In women, symptoms of chlamydia may include bleeding between menstrual periods, painful intercourse, vaginal bleeding after intercourse, swelling inside the vagina or around the anus, a yellowish discharge, and abdominal pain. If the disease results from oral sex, it can also cause a sore throat. In men, chlamydia symptoms include swollen or tender testicles, a pus or milky discharge from the penis, swelling around the anus, and pain or burning during urination. In some cases, chlamydia has no symptoms. Chlamydia can be easily treated with antibiotics, although if left untreated, it can lead to infertility in both men and women.

Trichomoniasis: Trichomoniasis, otherwise known as the "trich" (pronounced "trick"), is the most common curable STD in young, sexually active women. It is transmitted through intercourse, or through vulva-to-vulva contact with an infected partner. Women can acquire the disease from infected men or women, but men usually contract it only from infected women.

In women, the STD generally affects the vagina; in men, the urethra is the most common site of infection. Most men with trichomoniasis do not have signs or symptoms; however, some might notice a mild discharge, or slight burning after urination or ejaculation. In women, the

symptoms are much more evident. These include a frothy, yellow-green vaginal discharge with a strong odor, as well as pain during sex and urination. Itching and irritation might also occur. Trichomoniasis can be treated with antibiotics, but you can be re-infected following treatment.

Gonorrhea: Again, young people are at particular risk for this disease. In the US, almost 75 percent of all reported cases of gonorrhea are found in people who are 15–29 years of age. Like chlamydia, gonorrhea often has no symptoms. If symptoms are present in women, they might include abdominal pain, nausea, painful urination, swelling or tenderness of the vulva, a yellowish vaginal discharge, painful intercourse, and menstrual spotting. In men, symptoms of disease include pus-like discharge from the penis, frequent need to urinate, and pain during urination. Symptoms from oral sex

HOW TO ANSWER QUESTIONS ABOUT SEXUAL RISK

If your child asks a question that you don't know how to answer, promise to get back to him and then talk to a physician or research your answer online. Below are some of the most common questions the teens have about sexually transmitted diseases.

Q. Can I get an STD from kissing?
A. Yes. Some STDs can be transmitted through saliva or skin-to-skin contact. HIV can be present in saliva, though not in huge quantities, so it is unlikely to spread through kissing. However, HIV can enter through small cuts or sores around the mouth. Herpes and HPV can be spread through kissing.

Q. Do condoms always protect against STDs?
A. No. Even using a condom, you still have skin-to-skin contact with your partner around the genitals. STDs such as HPV and herpes can be spread when infected skin cells from one partner touch the other's skin.

Q. How can you tell if someone has an STD?
A. You can't rely on your eyes alone. STDs don't always have obvious symptoms like bumps or sores, although they sometimes do. Anyone can have an STD, even celebrities and popular kids. It is important that you always get an STD test before having sex with a new partner to make sure you are healthy. Your risk of contracting an STD increases as you have more partners, but you can still get an STD from one sexual encounter with just one sexual partner.

SEXPLANATION: **WHAT ARE THEY MYTHS AROUND PREGNANCY?**

Many teenagers do not have access to accurate sexual information. Indeed, most children grow up learning about sex from television or from what their friends or older siblings tell them, which is often wildly inaccurate. One recent survey in the United States found that 1 in 4 Florida teens believe that a shot of Mountain Dew can prevent pregnancy! Urban legends such as this might sound outrageous to adults, but to teens who are growing into their sexuality blindly, these legends are often all they have for guidance. Here are some of the most common myths teens buy into about sex and pregnancy:

• **Myth: You can't get pregnant if you have sex standing up.**
Truth: Sperm can travel to an egg regardless of the couple's position.

• **Myth: You can't get pregnant if you are on your period.**
Truth: Pregnancy is less likely when a woman is menstruating, but still highly possible because ovulation doesn't always occur at the same time during a woman's cycle.

• **Myth: If the guy pulls out, a girl can't get pregnant.**
Truth: Pre-ejaculate (the sperm which is ejaculated before a man reaches orgasm) is still capable of causing pregnancy. In addition, it is often hard for men to pull out in time, despite their best intentions to do so.

• **Myth: If you think you are pregnant, you can just take a bunch of birth control pills.**
Truth: Birth control pills do not affect an existing pregnancy. Furthermore, in order for birth control pills to be effective in preventing pregnancy, they generally need to taken very regularly—either at the same time or near the same time each day.

might include trouble swallowing or pain while swallowing—however, oral symptoms are rare. Additionally, gonorrhea symptoms might only occur in the morning, or might be most uncomfortable and prevalent in the morning. Gonorrhea can easily be treated with antibiotics, however, if left untreated, it can lead to infertility, stillbirth, or premature labor if the woman is pregnant, and to a disease known as disseminated gonococcal infection (DGI) which causes skin sores and arthritis. Gonorrhea can also cause serious eye infections.

Syphilis: Men are 3.5 times more likely to be diagnosed with syphilis than women. The disease has four stages: primary, secondary, latent, and tertiary. Antibiotics can cure syphilis at each stage, though if you wait too long to seek treatment, your physical and reproductive health can be damaged beyond repair.

In the primary stage, a sore (called a "chancre") appears on the body at the point of infection, whether oral, anal, or on the genitals. The sore is generally painless and will go away in a few weeks. However, if left untreated, the infection can move to the next stage.

During the secondary stage, skin rashes appear on the body, and are sometimes accompanied by itching. Other symptoms might include body ache, fever, weight loss, sore throat, and fatigue. Again, these symptoms will likely resolve themselves, but if left untreated, syphilis can move on to become latent, and can remain latent for years—sometimes symptoms of syphilis can appear up to 20 years after the infection was acquired. Syphilis can ultimately move on to the tertiary stage, and cause paralysis, numbness, gradual blindness, dementia. This stage can be fatal.

Herpes: Since the 1970s, the number of Americans with herpes (HSV-2) has increased by 30 percent. Indeed, 1 in 4 people have herpes, 80 percent of whom don't even know that they are infected. There are two types of herpes. One strain, HSV-1, is associated with common cold sores. The other strain, HSV-2, is similar and leads to painful sores in the oral and/or genital region. This strain also makes carriers more likely to contract other STDs, including HIV.

Herpes outbreaks are often accompanied by severe headaches and intense fatigue. Outbreaks generally appear as a red rash, sometimes progressing to blisters. Initial outbreaks are also sometimes associated with fevers and flu-like symptoms. Even if there are no visible lesions, herpes can be spread through a process known as shedding, in which the virus is active on the skin. Because a condom will not always cover the areas that are shedding, safer sex will not always protect against herpes.

Herpes cannot be cured, but its symptoms can be treated with medication. Medication can be taken daily (known as suppressive therapy), or it can be taken only when you feel an outbreak coming on (known as burst therapy). Burst therapy is often preferred because it reduces the amount of mediction required.

HIV/AIDS: More than 1 million people in the United States are infected with HIV/AIDS. Most new infections are found in men. In 2006, almost three quarters of HIV/AIDS diagnoses among adolescents and adults were for males. Men who have sex with men are the most likely to contract HIV/AIDS, followed by male heterosexuals who have high-risk sex. In addition, people under 25 years old account for half of all new HIV infections worldwide. HIV can remain asymptomatic for years. The earliest symptoms of the disease are similar to flu symptoms, such as fever, fatigue, and swollen glands. As HIV progresses and continues to attack the immune system, the body will begin to lose some of its ability to ward off infection, leading to symptoms such as chronic yeast infections, or thrush; yeast infection of the mouth; chronic diarrhea; extreme exhaustion; body rashes; fever; and easy bruising.

When HIV progresses to AIDS, a person can develop opportunistic infections, which prey upon a weakened immune system. These include Kaposi's Sarcoma, invasive cervical cancer, severe bacterial infections, recurrent pneumonia, and lymphoma. More than 25 million people have died of AIDS since 1981, but mortality rates have improved, particularly in the U.S.

There are now over 30 medications which can treat HIV. Antiretroviral drugs can help increase both the longevity and the quality of life of those infected with HIV/AIDS.

Pregnancy

Teenage pregnancy has been on the rise throughout the country in recent years. As a result, it is more important than ever to teach your child about contraception and the meaning of safer sex. Simply put, a teenager is not to ready to be a parent, and helping your child to understand this, as well as what this means for their sexual activity, is crucial.

Make this a constant conversation with your child—not a lecture, but a conversation. Each time you talk, be sure to stress the importance of using contraception during any sexual act. In addition to discussing the emotional and social costs of pregnancy (see pages 176–177), you might want to talk to your child about the actual financial expense of having a child, which can cost anywhere from $125,000 to $250,000 from birth to age 18. Explain that this added expense will mean no more nights at the movies or afternoons at the mall. It may seem superficial to bring up these types of leisurely consequences in relation to such a serious topic, but examples like these can help your child to picture the realities of this substantial risk to sexual and emotional health.

Teaching about sexual protection

One reason parents choose not to talk to their children about safer sex is because they fear doing so will give permission to become sexually active. It is good to use abstinence as your family's central value, but neglecting to give any further information can be dangerous. Teaching about contraception will help ensure that if your child does have sex, it will be the safest experience possible.

Abstinence

There are two schools of thought when it comes to sexual education. Abstinence-only education is when adolescents are taught only that sex is dangerous and can cause disease and pregnancy, and thus should be avoided until marriage or adulthood. There is no discussion of safer sex or birth control. In abstinence-based education, adolescents are taught that sex can be dangerous, that every sexual experience has the potential to cause both STD transmission and pregnancy, but that safer sex practices (such as using condoms) can help to protect against these. Abstinence is put forward as the best option, for both physical and emotional reasons, but teens are taught how sex works and how to use condoms in order to be safe if they do decide not to wait.

Research has shown that while abstinence-only education might delay a child's initiation into sexual activity, it only does so for a short time. A study published in the United States in April 2009 found that teens who received abstinence-based sex education were 50% less likely to become pregnant than those who received abstinence-only education, and 60% less likely to become pregnant than teens who received no sex education at all. Thus, by failing to educate your child about contraception, you may be failing to provide the support your child needs to make smart sexual decisions. If you are worried that giving your teenager information about safer sex will cause her to be sexual, you can incorporate that into your talks with her. **For example, you might say:** "I want you to know that I am not giving information about condoms and birth control because I think that you are ready to have sex. I absolutely don't think you are ready for such a big step. But I want you to have the information you need to be safe just in case you do decide to have sex. Remember that even though this information will help you to be safe physically, it can't keep you safe emotionally. In addition, even using protection doesn't make sex 100% safe—that's why we call it safer sex, not safe sex."

Protection during alternate sex play

When talking about safer sex practices, it is important to talk about how protection is necessary during oral and anal sex. While you might feel uncomfortable addressing these topics with your child, remember that his safety is more important than your own discomfort. Oral and anal sex are increasingly common among teenagers, due to the lack of risk of pregnancy and because many teens don't think of them as "sex" in the same way they think of intercourse as sex. It is important to talk about these topics with your child, and to stress that all of these sexual activities are sexual acts.

SEXPLANATION
WHAT TYPES OF CONTRACEPTION ARE AVAILABLE?

Make sure your child knows the benefits and disadvantages of each type of contraception available. Hold this conversation at a time when there won't be any distractions so that your child can process the information and ask questions. Start by saying that you want to build upon the discussions you've had in the past by sharing crucial information about sexual health.

METHOD OF PROTECTION	EFFECTIVENESS
THE CONDOM is a barrier method of contraception that traps sperm. The male condom fits over the penis in a latex sheath. The less commonly used female condom is made of polyurethane, and is inserted deep into the vagina just before intercourse.	Used correctly, a condom is 98 percent effective in preventing pregnancy. Putting the condom on midway through intercourse will reduce its level of protection, as will using oil-based lubricants, which can damage latex. Condoms offer the best protection against STDs, aside from abstinence.
THE CONTRACEPTIVE INJECTION releases the hormone progestin, preventing ovulation, and thickening the cervical mucous to block sperm. Injections are effective for three months.	A contraceptive injection offers 99 percent protection against pregnancy. It is most effective when injected every 12 weeks. It does not provide any protection against STDs.
THE IUD, or intrauterine device, comes in hormonal and non-hormonal form. The T-shaped copper device works by preventing sperm from reaching the fallopian tubes. It also alters the lining of the uterus so it is uninhabitable for a fertilized egg. It will stay in place for 5–12 years.	The intrauterine device is convenient and effective, offering 99 percent protection against pregnancy. However, it does not protect against STDs. In fact, the IUD may even act as a dangerous viaduct for STDs, allowing a virus to spread directly up to the cervix.
THE ORAL CONTRACEPTIVE PILL consists of estrogen and progesterone, which act together to prevent ovulation so that fertilization cannot occur. Side-effects can include weight gain, headaches, and decreased sex drive.	The pill has a 99 percent rate of preventing pregnancy when taken properly, but offers no protection against STDs. Many types must be taken at the same time every day so that hormone levels in the body remain the same.
THE DIAPHRAGM is a rubber disc that can be put in place in the vagina just before intercourse or 2–3 hours beforehand. Post-intercourse, it must be left in for 6–8 hours. The diaphragm must be used with spermicide, a jelly or cream that destroys sperm, to effectively impede pregnancy.	The diaphragm is 85–94 percent effective in preventing pregnancy, though it can be difficult to use correctly. To ensure that it is most effective, it is essential that it covers the cervix and that spermicide is used. The diaphragm does not protect against STDs.
THE FLEXIBLE CONTRACEPTIVE RING contains hormones that are absorbed into the vaginal lining and bloodstream. It is inserted into the vagina each month.	The vaginal ring is 99 percent effective when inserted properly. It works best when it is kept in place for three weeks, then removed for the fourth week. It does not protect against STDs.

Often teens think that oral sex has fewer consequences than actual intercourse, but the truth is that this act of intimacy can transmit STDs just as easily as intercourse—if not more so, as saliva and other bodily fluids are being exchanged. Because of this, protection is always a must when engaging in oral sex. Young men should use condoms, and young women should use dental dams, which are placed around the vulva during oral sex to prevent the transmission of saliva into the genital area. Dental dams can be found in most drugstores that offer safer sex products. They are also often available at family planning clinics or at your doctor's office. If a dental dam is not available, saran wrap can be used to help prevent the exchange of fluids, although this can be more difficult to keep in place.

Although you might think that it should go without saying, it is important to tell your teen to use protection during anal sex as well. Anal sex can't lead to pregnancy, and for this reason, many teens think it is safe to engage in this activity without protection. Indeed, some people still consider themselves virgins after anal sex, despite how intimate this act is. It is important to let your child know that anal sex can still transmit STDs and that a condom should be used every time you engage in this type of intimacy. **To broach this topic with your child,** you might say something like, "I have to admit this is a little uncomfortable to talk about, but I still want to have this conversation because your health is the most important thing to me. I want you to know that every type of sexual activity comes with risk, and this is why I want you to be abstinent. But if you choose not to be, or if you engage in non-vaginal sex, like oral sex or anal sex, remember that you still need to use protection every time."

Obtaining contraception

If you think your child may be engaging in sexual activity, or is likely to engage in sexual activity in the near future, it is a good idea to mention specifics about how to get contraception, or even to provide that contraception yourself. You can be very clear about your desires for your child not to engage in sexual activity even as you are passing along contraception information. For example, try reiterating your safer sex talk as you provide condoms or another form of protection. If you have a daughter, you might consider giving her birth control pills or encouraging her to talk about contraception with her ob/gyn, but don't forget to tell her that not all contraceptives prevent STDs. If you don't feel comfortable providing protection yourself, remind your child about safer sex as you tell her that a variety of types of protection are available at your local family planning clinic, or at your doctor's office. **For example, you might say,** "I am not giving you contraception because I think that you are ready to have sex or because I want you to have sex. Instead, I am doing this because I want to make sure you have all the resources and information you need to make safer sexual decisions in every circumstance."

"You can be very clear about your desires for your child not to engage in sexual activity even as you are passing along contraception information."

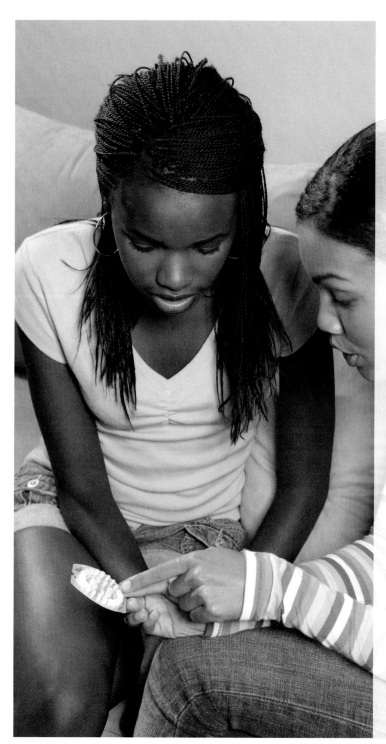

WHAT TO SAY . . .
IF YOU THINK YOUR CHILD MIGHT NEED CONTRACEPTION

If you think your child is engaging in sexual activity, or is planning to engage in sexual activity in the near future, sit down and talk with her. During this talk, you can reassert your family values about when it is appropriate to start having sex.

CONVERSATION STARTER: "We have talked about how important it is to wait to have sex until you are older. But, in the end, only you can make that decision."

You can then go on to express your opinion about her decision to have sex, and elaborate on how important it is to use contraception.

FOLLOW-UP: "While I don't support your decision to have sex at such a young age, I want you to have all the information and the tools you need. There is no such thing as safe sex—but if you use condoms every time, you can help protect yourself against STDs and pregnancy."

Give your child a chance to respond, then remind her exactly why it is that you are giving her protection. Stress that this is not a permissive action, and that you do not think she is making the most responsible choice, but that you still want to protect and support her.

FOLLOW-UP: "The reason I am giving you condoms isn't because I want you to have sex. I am not giving you permission to take this step, but I do want you to be as safe as possible, even when you are making decisions that I don't agree with."

Learning together

LEARNING ABOUT USING CONTRACEPTION

Some methods of contraception are more straightforward to use than others. Long-acting types, such as the contraceptive injection, do not depend upon your child remembering to take them or use them properly. With short-acting methods, such as the diaphragm, oral contraceptive pill, and condoms, correct usage is essential if they are to be effective. Once your child reaches her teens, talk her through the practicalities of using contraception, especially condoms, which, for girls, should ideally be used in conjunction with another form of birth control to protect against both pregnancy and STDs.

....

AFTER THIS LESSON YOUR CHILD WILL BE MORE LIKELY TO...
- Feel confident about talking about contraception and safer sex
- Understand that there are no excuses not to use condoms
- Be able to put on a condom properly
- Make the sensible choice to use two types of protection
- Have a clearer idea of which form of contraception might be most suitable

....

1 WHAT'S RELIABLE AND EASIEST TO USE?

You may want to reiterate to your teen that no single method is 100 percent safe, but that using a condom and one other form of protection consistently and responsibly is the most effective way to guard against pregnancy and infection. The oral contraceptive pill, the contraceptive patch, or the new vaginal ring—used with a condom—are highly effective methods and among the easiest to use. The pill does need to be taken every day, however, and generally at the same time of day. Is your child likely to remember to do this? Explain that if she misses a dose, she will need to use a back-up form of protection for the rest of her cycle. The diaphragm, cap, and sponge have a higher rate of failure than other methods. Let your teen know that these can take a while to get used to, but are easy to use once learned, so not to get frustrated. Allow your child the freedom to choose whatever method she is comfortable with, then stress the importance of using it each and every time.

2 WHAT ARE THE EXCUSES FOR NOT USING CONDOMS AS A FORM OF PROTECTION?

One of the most common complaints about condoms is that they ruin the mood. Some say that having to stop, search for a condom, and put one on is a passion killer. Stress to your teen that this need not be the case if condoms are kept easily accessible. There are ways to put condoms on that are fun and sexy, especially if the woman does it. Another excuse is that they reduce sensation. Condoms do make sex feel different, but not less enjoyable. In fact, many condoms have features such as ribbing, which can make sex more pleasurable. It is also helpful to put some water-based lubricant in the tip of the condom to increase sensation. There are also those who think condoms are a waste of time if neither they nor their partners have an STD. But sometimes STDs don't have any symptoms for years, so you might not know if you have one. The bottom line is that it is important to always use condoms to stay safe.

3 WHAT IS EMERGENCY CONTRACEPTION?

Your teen needs to know that emergency contraception is a way to prevent pregnancy after unprotected sex. Often called the morning-after pill, emergency contraceptive pills can be taken up to 72 hours after unprotected sex. However, the sooner you take the pill, the more effective it is. Stress that ECPs are not a regular method of birth control and do not protect against STDs.

PUTTING ON A CONDOM

1. CHECKING THE CONDOM IS INTACT

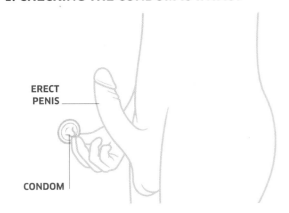

ERECT PENIS

CONDOM

Carefully take the condom out of its packaging and check that it is not brittle, stiff, or sticky. If it is, throw it away and use another. The penis has to be hard before putting on a condom. (If the penis is not circumcised, pull back the foreskin.)

2. POSITIONING THE CONDOM

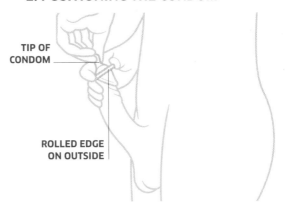

TIP OF CONDOM

ROLLED EDGE ON OUTSIDE

Place the rolled up condom on the tip of the penis, with the brim on the outside. Leave about a half-inch of space in the tip. Pinch out the air in the tip of the sheath. Putting some water-based lubricant in the tip of the condom will help to increase sensation.

3. ROLLING THE CONDOM DOWN

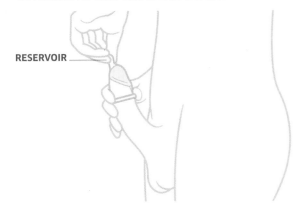

RESERVOIR

Carefully unroll the condom down the penis with one hand while pinching the tip with the other. It's essential to leave a reservoir at the tip to collect the semen. If you don't pinch the top it can fill with air and be more likely to break during ejaculation.

4. ENSURING THE CONDOM IS SECURE

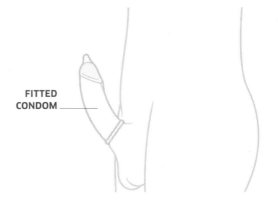

FITTED CONDOM

Unroll the condom all the way to the base of the penis. Check that it fits snugly and does not feel loose, or it may slip during intercourse. After sex, carefully remove the condom from the penis while it's still erect. Then throw the condom away.

Learning together

Making sexual decisions

Although you cannot make sexual decisions for your child, your guidance can have a huge impact on your child's decisions. Staying involved in your child's social life will allow you to help your child work through peer pressure situations, examine sexual motivations, and think about the ramifications of increasingly popular types of teenage sexual activity like oral and anal sex.

Dealing with peer pressure

Part of the reason that teenagers, especially teenage girls, find it hard to make wise sexual decisions is because they want to be popular. Many young girls believe that the girl who gives the most sexually will attract the most male attention, and that this will make her more popular with the girls as well. It is a good idea to talk about this directly with your child, and remind her that while this might be true for a short while, the attention only lasts as long as the act itself. So, while another girl might get more attention for being sexually active, the attention is purely physical, and will not be satisfying in the long-term. You can also inform her of a recent poll in "Perspectives on Sexual and Reproductive Health" which found that almost a third of teenagers regret the first time they had sex, and that 19 percent of girls reported feeling pressured into their first sexual experience.

Boys are under a lot of pressure as well. They are expected to always be ready for sex. When girls act sexually assertive, boys can receive the same level of judgment from their peers if they don't pursue sexual opportunities.

Empowering your teen to say "no" and providing the tools to do so can encourage the right decisions when she faces difficult decisions like these. Talking openly about the challenges of sexual peer pressure is the best way to do this. For example, let your child know that anyone who pressures her to have sex does not have her best interests at heart. Troubleshoot possible situations that might occur, such as a boyfriend who says she doesn't love him if she won't sleep with him, or a girl offering a sexual encounter and his peers pressuring him to accept or be deemed homosexual or lame. **Help your child think of possible responses** to these situations, whether it's deciding to walk away or saying something like, "If you really loved me, you would not pressure me to have sex before I am ready. I am going to wait to have sex until I am [married, older, etc.] If you aren't comfortable waiting, then this isn't going to work," or "I'm very interested in your offer but I usually don't do that unless I have a really strong connection with the girl, and I don't think we have that." Encourage your child to find positive, proactive ways to deal with the the temptation of peer pressure, and you can help foster smart decisions, sexually and otherwise.

Examining sexual motivations

Ultimately, you can't prevent your child from choosing his own sexual path, but you can play a role in helping him think about why he wants to have sex. If your child expresses that he feels ready for sex, or if you notice other indicators

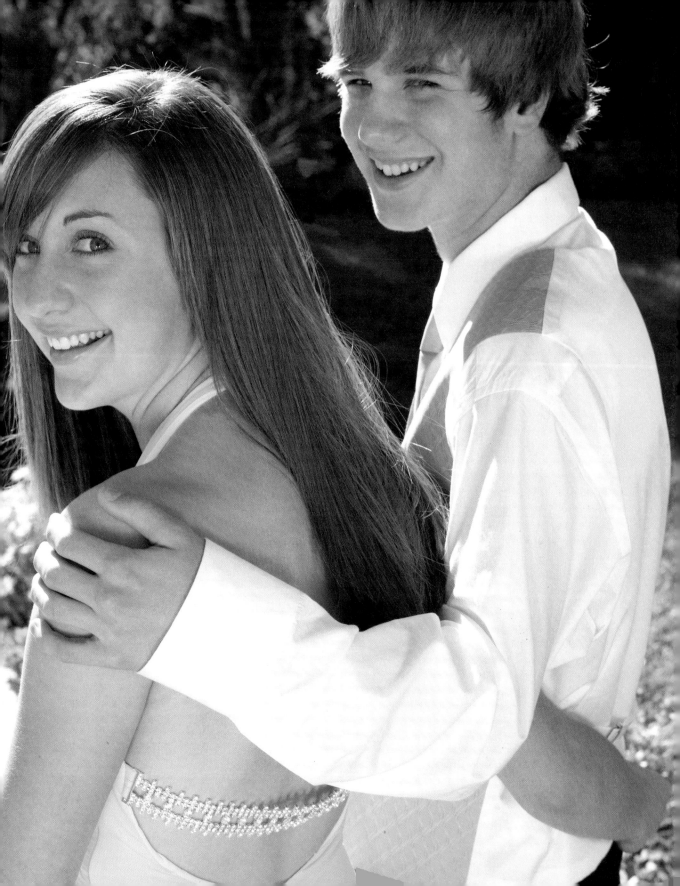

that his relationship is getting more physically intimate, ask him about his motivation to try sex for the first time. Is it because he is curious, because he thinks he is ready to take that next step in his relationship, because he wants to fit in with the other kids at school, or because he thinks it will feel good? Although your child might act annoyed that you are questioning his motivation, it may help to spark some self-introspection that can help him to discover whether he is ready to make this big decision.

When it comes to sexual decisions, most teens—and even many adults—don't spend very much time examining their reasoning. Encourage your child to look inward and see what is driving him toward sexual activity. If hormones or physical pleasure are the driving force, remind him that self-stimulation can help release some of that tension and help to postpone sexual activity until he is a little older.

For example, you might say, "Sexual feelings and thoughts are part of growing up, and right now, you are experiencing a wave of these feelings for the first time. However, you don't have to rush into sex in order to release those feelings and explore your sexuality. Masturbation is a way that a lot of teens and adults release that sexual tension until a time when they are ready to be intimate with their significant other."

If he is feeling pressured from his friends, inform him that many of the people he hears bragging about sex in the locker room are not telling the truth. You might talk about how the very fact that these kids are always talking about sex is proof that they aren't mature enough to handle the responsibility that comes with being intimate.

Try saying something such as: "I know that a lot of kids your age are probably talking about sex, and that some of them are even talking about their sexual experiences. But, it's good to keep in mind that a lot of those stories probably aren't true. Even if they are, you shouldn't rush into

sex at a young age just because other kids are. It is so much better to wait to have sex until you are [in a committed relationship, an adult, married, etc.], when it will be meaningful and feel good."

Talking about oral and anal sex

A study released by the National Center for Health Statistics found that almost half of all American teens aged 15-19 have engaged in oral sex. The number increases the older teens are, and about 70% of teens aged 18-19 have done so. The same study found that 4.6 percent of 15-year-old boys have had anal sex with a female—the number jumps to 34 percent by the ages of 22-24. And, by age 24, 1 in 3 women has tried anal sex.

Clearly, sexual education cannot begin and end with the discussion of traditional intercourse, especially because many of these sexual encounters do not involve protection. A study published in the "Journal of Pediatric Phsycology" found that 70% of teenagers do not use protection during oral sex, and that these teens have multiple oral sex partners. 23% of teens responded that they had been with three to four oral sex partners within the last year. For most teens, oral sex is seen as much less intimate and risky than intercourse, since it carries with it no risk of pregnancy and is seen as preserving one's virginity. In other words, many teens view oral sex as "third base" on the way to "home plate" and intercourse. However, as far as STDs go, unprotected oral sex is as risky as unprotected intercourse, and it is equally risky from an emotional standpoint. This is especially true for young girls. For most of these girls, giving oral sex is a way of currying favor or acceptance from boys—yet, once the incident is over, the boy might never talk to the girl again, or might tell other kids at school about the experience. Because of this, it is important to talk to both girls and boys about the concept of giving oral sex, and how it is meant to be shared in a loving, committed relationship, with a give-and-take philosophy.

For instance, you might say to your daughter: "You know I heard on the news the other day that oral sex is becoming more common among junior high and high school students. The sad part is that oral sex is just as intimate as intercourse, but kids seem to treat it as casually as they do kissing. It especially makes me sad to think about young girls performing oral sex on boys in order to be accepted. I hope you know that you don't have to perform oral sex in order make boys like you, and that your body is much too valuable to be treated with such disrespect. What do you think about girls giving boys oral sex? Is that something you hear about in your school a lot? Do boys give oral sex to girls too, or is that not part of the deal?"

You might also say to your teenage son: "I hear a lot about young girls giving boys oral sex these days, but I don't hear a lot about boys doing the same. I know you are respectful of women and you wouldn't ever use them for a sexual purpose, but do you have friends that talk about oral sex like that? Do they think oral sex involves give-and-take, or do they just expect girls to do it?"

It might seem a little strange to talk to your teen about the importance of viewing sex as a give-and-take exchange, but you want to help your teen to learn to respect his partner and to view pleasure as something that should always be shared. The more that your teen views sex as something that is meant to be special and pleasurable for both people, the less likely he will be to try to use sex as a means to an end and the less likely he will be to engage in casual or promiscuous sex. This is also a good time to talk to your teenager about the fact that everyone has different boundaries and sexual expectations, and that while he might be ready to engage in sexual activities, his partner might not be ready for this step. Teach your child to respect a partner's wish for abstinence and to never pressure or goad her into having sex, including oral sex.

TEACHABLE MOMENT
TALKING ABOUT ORAL SEX

There are plenty of media moments that will give you a chance to discuss oral sex with your child, whether it is a new study that has found that more teens are having oral sex, or a story about a celebrity who was filmed in the act. Use these moments to teach your teen about the potential risks of oral sex, by saying something such as, "Did you hear the story about those teens that were caught having oral sex at school? Many people don't realize that oral sex is just as dangerous as intercourse, as far as the transmission of STDs goes. Even though you can't get pregnant from oral sex, you can contract an STD, including herpes, HIV, or Chlamydia."

CONVERSATION STARTER 1: "Is oral sex common at your school? It may seem safer than intercourse, but in reality, having casual oral sex can be just as damaging as having casual intercourse."

CONVERSATION STARTER 2: "Did you hear about that celebrity video that showed [insert celebrity names here] performing oral sex? It is so sad that such a private moment was caught on video. It is also very dangerous for them to be engaging in such intimate acts together, especially when it is a new relationship, and they may not know each other's sexual histories."

Encouraging healthy sexual decisions

The ultimate goal of sex education should not be to convince your child not to have sex, but to guide him to wait until sexual intimacy is meaningful, safe, and pleasurable—whatever that means in the context of your personal family values. Encourage your child to set personal sexual goals that reflect the value of his sexuality, his identity, and his relationships.

Setting personal sexual goals

Most teenagers make sexual decisions without any pre-planning. An ABC News poll found that 70 percent of teens admitted their first time was unplanned. A lack of forethought often means a lack of protection, which means safer sex was not practiced. These impulsive decisions often result in regret: Another survey found that 90% of girls under the age of 16 regret their first sexual experience.

Talk to your teen about these statistics, and about how she envisions her first time to be. This conversation doesn't have to be too graphic. Simply ask your child about what hopes she has for her first sexual experience: How old does she want to be? What type of relationship does she want to be in? By discussing her sexual goals the same way you would talk to her about any of her other goals, you can help her to understand that she is in control of her sexual experiences and that she has can create the outcome she desires. Helping your child plan specific goals for how and when she loses her virginity can prevent her first sexual experience from being unplanned and regrettable.

For example, you might say, "Have you ever thought about how you would like your first time to be? Do you know where you want to be and who you want to be with? It's okay to think about stuff like that—in fact, it is important. Planning your sexual goals is part of being a healthy adult. While you might not know everything about how you want your first time

>>> **YOUR CHILD IS IN A HEALTHY RELATIONSHIP IF . . .**

While it is often easy to tell when your child is making bad decisions within her relationships, it can be harder to tell when she is making a healthy choice and when you can be confident in these choices. Generally speaking, a child in a healthy relationship will be happy and relaxed about the relationship. Some signs include:
• Greater confidence and a more relaxed and easygoing attitude
• Increasing signs of maturity, such as becoming more vigilant about keeping a curfew
• Acting more selflessly, perhaps by being more willing to take care of younger siblings or help out around the house
• Becoming more goal-oriented in school, sports, or other activities

be, you can have a list of certain "must haves"–such as you must be with someone you love, you must be somewhere private and romantic, you must have protection."

Sharing sexual history

When discussing sexual goals and sexual planning with your teenagers, you might run into some questions about your own past sexual decisions. Answering these questions can sometimes be tricky, because you don't want your teenager to think it's okay to make certain mistakes just because you have made them.

A good rule of thumb is not to bring up your own sexual past unless your child directly questions you. If your child does confront you about your sexual past, use your own judgment to decide if he is mature enough to have this conversation. If not, you can tell your child that it is a discussion for a later date. If you do think that he is mature enough to handle the

information, fill him in with just the bare facts, and don't be too detailed. It is a good idea to focus on any lessons that you learned from these experiences, rather than specific details of how and when the experience occurred.

For example, you might say: "I started having sex too young. My parents never talked about sex, condoms, or anything like that with me, so I had to find my own way. As a result, I think I took a lot of risks I shouldn't have and I also missed out on having a special first experience. I wish I could go back now and take back some of those early mistakes. Instead, I am hoping to give you all the support and information you need so that you don't make my same mistakes."

If your teen does have a lot of questions for you about your own sexual past, ask him why this is. It could be because he is being confronted with sexual decisions of his own, or because he has questions or concerns that he wants to talk about. Talk to him about what is driving these questions and offer your support.

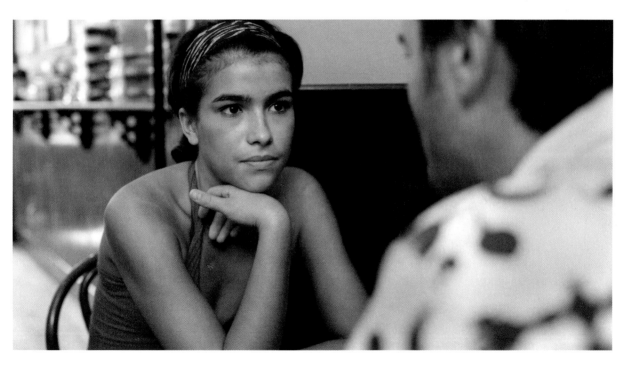

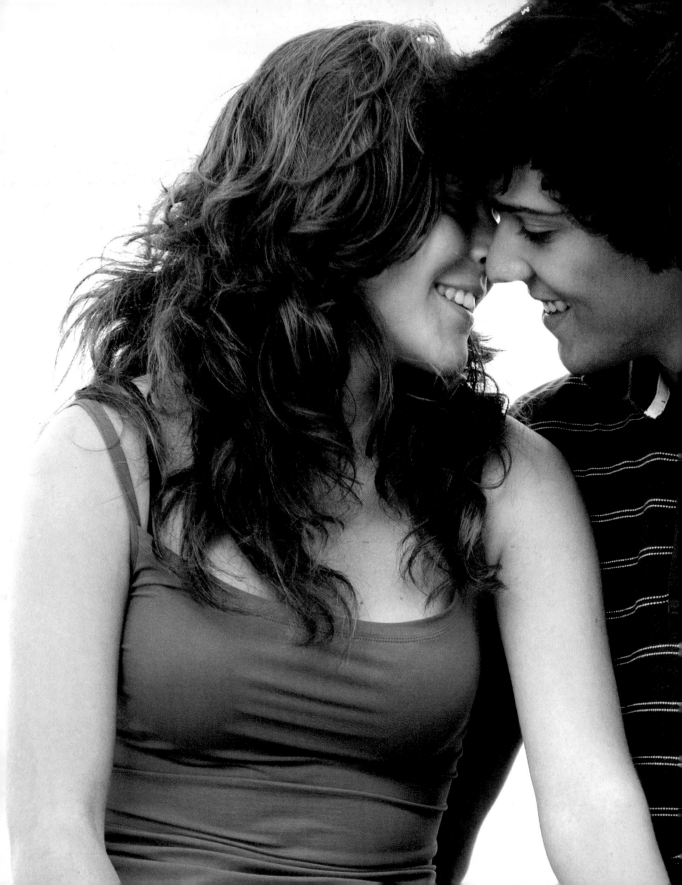

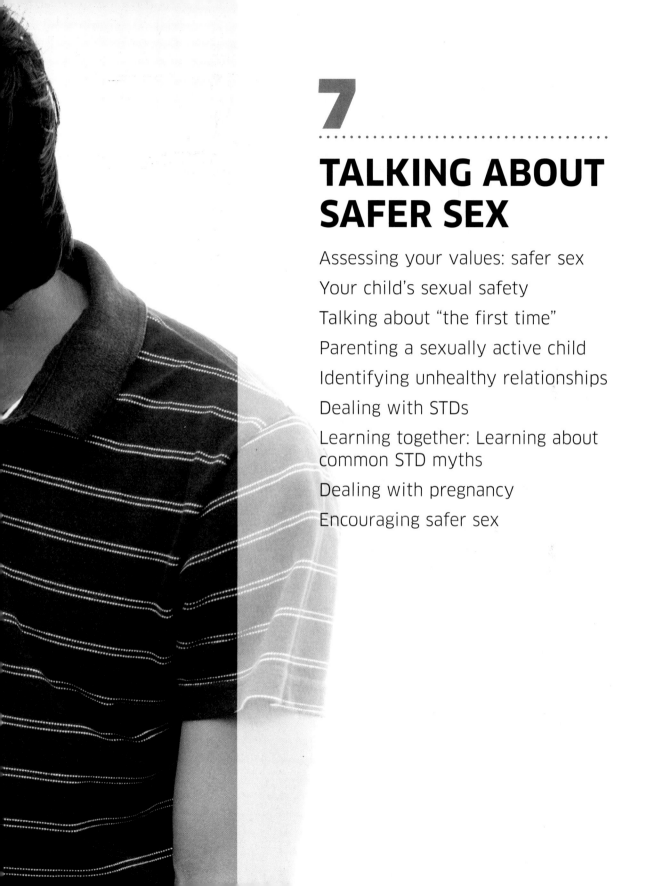

7

TALKING ABOUT SAFER SEX

ASSESSING YOUR VALUES: SAFER SEX

The final mile in raising a sexually healthy child is teaching about safer sex. There is no such thing as "safe sex," other than no sex. Helping your child understand that every sexual decision has a consequence—either physical or emotional or both—will go a long way in helping him grasp the gravity of sexual activity. Before you can teach these important lessons, however, take time to reflect on your own values. Consider the following questions privately, then discuss them with your partner.

EXPLORING SEXUAL COMMUNICATION

Communicating clearly about sex—both your own history and your child's experience—is an important parenting tool. Reflect on these questions to decide how involved you want to be as your child moves toward greater intimacy.

If your child asks you about your own sexual history (e.g. when you first had sex, what the experience was like), how much information do you feel is appropriate to share?

If you know your child is sexually active, do you think you have a responsibility to tell his partner's parents?

How involved do you think you should be if you feel your child is in an unhealthy relationship?

How would you support your child if he chose to become sexually active?

EXPLORING SEXUAL DECISIONS

Think about what goes into a wise sexual decision, and what values you want your child to consider as she begins making her own decisions about sex.

What signs of emotional maturity do you think are necessary before entering into a sexual relationship?

What signs of relationship maturity are necessary in order to create a healthy environment for sex?

How much do you value monogamy?

What would you say if your child was in a healthy relationship and felt she was ready to have sex? Would this change based on age?

How would you react if your child was in an unhealthy relationship and felt ready for this big commitment?

How much of a role do you think you should play in your child's decision-making process?

EXPLORING SEXUAL HEALTH

Communicating clearly about healthy sexuality can help protect your child against obvious dangers, such as STDs, and less obvious ones, such as emotional pain.

What do you think are the characteristics of an emotionally unhealthy relationship?

What are the characteristics of a physically unhealthy relationship?

How will you react if your child confides in you that she had a bad sexual experience—or even a forced sexual experience?

Do you know about the most common STDs, including how they are transmitted and treated?

Have you ever been tested for an STD?

What are you beliefs about STD prevention?

How much information do you want to communicate to your child about STDs, and at what age do you think you should begin having this conversation?

EXPLORING SEXUAL CONSEQUENCES

Although hopefully your family will not be exposed to the potentially negative consequences of teenage sex, it is a good idea to think about how you would react if your child were to become pregnant or contact an STD, and in what ways you would be able to support your child.

Do you think it is important to address the realities of sexual consequences (e.g. STDs, pregnancy, etc.) with your child in advance?

What are your thoughts on teenage pregnancy?

How do you think teenage pregnancy can be prevented?

How would you react if your teen confessed she was pregnant?

If your teen was pregnant, what options would you encourage her to consider (e.g. abortion, adoption, raising the baby herself)? What would you do if she chose an option that you didn't agree with, or thought was morally wrong?

What are your views on abortion?

How would you react if your teen confessed he had an STD?

APPLYING YOUR ANSWERS As you reflect on these questions, you might feel anxious or overwhelmed at the thought of introducing your child to such harsh realities. Remember that this information can give your child the knowledge and emotional support he needs to make smart sexual decisions. When it comes to information about safer sex practices, silence can be deadly. If you find it difficult to agree on any of these questions, consider asking a trusted friend or mentor to help you reach a decision, so that you can present a united front to your child.

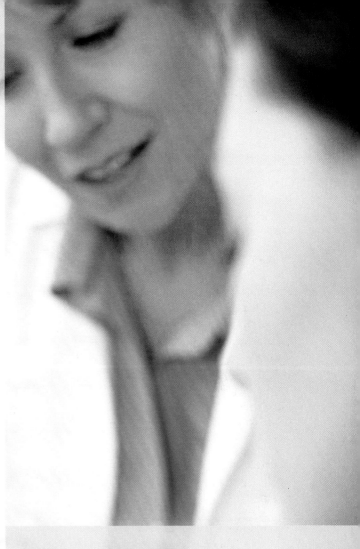

Your child's sexual safety

In addition to your family values about sex, there are two primary factors that impact whether or not your child might be ready for greater intimacy—emotional maturity and relationship maturity. As your child's relationship becomes more serious, hold frequent conversations with her. The more you understand about your child, the better you will be able to protect against unsound decisions.

Your child's emotional maturity

An important part of sexual safety is making sure you are able to handle the emotional commitment that comes with an intimate relationship. This is especially true for teenagers, who may not have made this level of emotional commitment before. However, judging the emotional maturity of a growing adolescent can be difficult. Adolescence truly is a balancing act of childhood and adulthood, so it is no wonder that emotional maturity seems to present itself in spurts that are difficult to gauge.

For this reason, parenting a teen can be a bit of a balancing act in and of itself. There is no set time when your child will be ready to start making healthy sexual decisions or relationship decisions. The only way to truly monitor your child's behavior in an age-appropriate manner is to stay aware of what is going on in her life. Talk to your child about the decisions her friends are making and about how they are managing the sometimes tricky world of relationships. Ask her if she feels ready to have a serious boyfriend or if she thinks she is ready to have sex. Talk about why she feels this way and if she has any fears or anxieties about getting older and making these adult decisions.

Indicators that she may be ready to make emotionally mature commitments include: a willingness to respect your point of view; an ability to understand the many potential consequences of sexual activity; and the development of personal sexual goals. In other

>>> YOUR CHILD MAY BE READY FOR SEX WHEN...

Scary though it may seem, one day your child will be ready to have sex. When this is depends largely on your family values, and what age or relationship situation you think is appropriate for such an intimate step. Character signs that indicate your child may be responsible enough to take this step include:
• Being responsible for adult decisions in other areas of life (e.g. by paying a car payment, working hard towards a goal, etc.)
• Acting respectful toward the opposite sex and toward sexuality in general
• Valuing the needs of a significant other, and working or making sacrifices to maintain a happy, secure relationship

words, an emotionally mature teenager does not make sexual decisions without forethought, or to please others. Instead, sex is a way to enjoy intimacy with her partner and to engage in the give-and-take of pleasure. Hormones will stay play a part, but her decision to have sex is based on thoughtful, consideration.

Your child's relationship maturity

It isn't always easy to know what is going on in your child's relationship, especially because as things become more serious, he might want privacy and thus seek to shut you out. However, if you have previously established an open conversation with your child about sex and relationships, you can continue to talk about this in the context of your child's relationship.

If you haven't had this discussion yet, begin by reaching out to your child and showing an interest in his relationship. Try to communicate with a lack of judgment and with an understanding, accepting attitude. Put effort into getting to know your child's partner, and make room in your home and family to include and accept this important part of your child's life. Ask your child questions and seek out his thoughts about the relationship. If your child doesn't feel judged, he will be less likely to be defensive and more likely to open up to you and want to share his life with you.

Find a time when you and your child can talk privately, such as while you are driving in the car together, or while you are browsing at the mall. Bring up the conversation in a non-judgmental way, and instead, just show your interest in his life and his relationship. **You might try saying something like,** "You seem very happy with Alisha. I am glad you found someone who you care about so much. Tell me more about her again. What was the first thing that you noticed about her? Did you like her right away, or did it develop over time?"

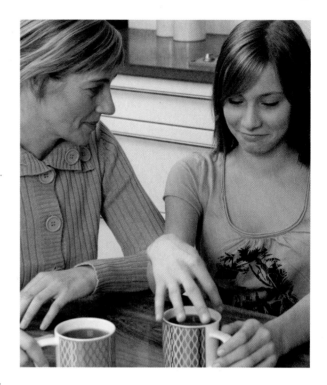

Your child might laugh and act indifferent about your interest, but on the inside he will be pleased that you are talking to him about the relationship like an adult. This will help him feel more comfortable sharing details of the relationship with you—including whether he and his partner have discussed taking their relationship to the next level physically.

As you talk with your child, listen for signs that his relationship is stable enough to support sexual intimacy. Indications of this might include: a mutual respect for each other's needs and desires, both sexually and otherwise; maintaining an open discussion about contraception and safer sex; an openness to regular STD testing and other sexual health precautions; and a commitment to practicing honesty, trust, and open communication. If your child's relationship seems to exhibit these traits, both partners are more likely to be able to deal with the emotional implications of sex.

Talking about "the first time"

Perhaps the most important talk you will have with your child about sex is when you think he is about to become sexually active. If you keep an open atmosphere at home, your child may feel comfortable talking with you before this milestone event. In fact, it is a good idea to encourage him to do so, in order to make sure that he is prepared and has thought through his choice carefully.

Encouraging your child to open up

One of the best ways to help your child make smart sexual decisions is to begin the conversation before she starts making them. Have a policy that she can always talk to you about sexual decisions without fear of repercussion or punishment.

For example, you might say something like: "I know that you and your boyfriend have been together for a while. I also know that relationships and sex sometimes go hand-in-hand, even at your age. While I don't think you are ready to have sex, I know that the decision is ultimately your own. However, I do ask that you think about coming to me before you decide to have sex for the first time. I want to make sure you have all the information and protection you need before you have sex. In return, while I may not be happy and may not approve, I promise not to judge you or get angry with you."

Having a conversation like this is a positive, protective measure against unsafe sexual decisions. When your child is empowered to make her own decisions and feels responsible for her own sexual destiny, she will be more likely to make choices that are based on values, not on physical temptation. Whether or not these choices involve waiting, you can be comforted in knowing that you have left the door open for her to talk with you.

The pre-sex talk

If your child does come to you, ask about his motivations for having sex, and how he knows that this is the right time. Ask questions about his frame of mind, his partner's, and their future plans for the relationship. Discussing these questions in a non-judgmental way will help guide your child through the decision-making process. The idea is to play devil's advocate in a loving and supportive way that will encourage your child to weigh the consequences and realities of the choices he is making without causing him to seek to rebel.

To start this conversation, try saying: "I am so proud of you for being honest about the fact that you think you are ready to have sex. Can I ask you a couple of questions, though? What is it about this person and this relationship that makes you feel she deserves such an amazing gift? What have you discussed about the future of your relationship? Will you get tested for STDs? What kind of protection will you use? Do you know how to use a condom? Have you talked about what will happen if she gets pregnant? Have you discussed whether your sexual activity will be private or whether you will discuss it with friends?" Questions like these can serve as a pre-sex "checklist" for you child, and will also remind him of the responsibilities that come with sex in a non-alienating way.

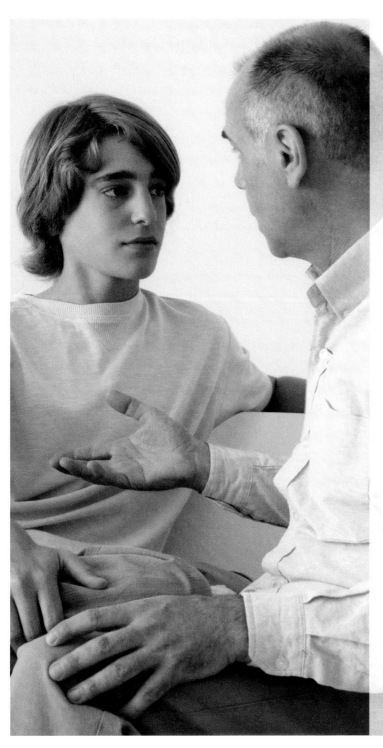

WHAT TO SAY IF . . .
YOU DON'T THINK YOUR CHILD IS READY FOR SEX

If you find out your child is planning to have sex, it is important to have a direct, open, and non-judgmental conversation. This is true even if you feel strongly that your child is not ready to take this step.

CONVERSATION STARTER: "I know that you are feeling pressure from a lot of different people in your life to have sex–possibly even your friends and your girlfriend.

After introducing the topic, legitimize your child's natural desires.

FOLLOW-UP: "It is okay to want to have sex–your adult body was built to have sexual desires, and you are growing into that body as we speak."

Begin to insert your own values into the conversation, stressing what a big responsibility it is to have sex.

FOLLOW-UP: "Still, I think it's important that you don't act on those sexual feelings before you are ready to handle the potential consequences of those decisions. I want you to have a happy sex life someday, and if you have sex too soon, that can make future relationships very difficult.

Close with an attitude of openness, so that your teen doesn't feel judged.

FOLLOW-UP: "I can't make this decision for you, but I just ask that you spend plenty of time thinking about it. Don't rely on your friends' opinions or base your decisions on what other people are doing. You are the only person who can protect your body and your sexuality."

Parenting a sexually active child

If your child becomes sexually active, it can easily and sometimes dramatically alter your relationship, especially if you disagree with her decisions. The most effective way to influence your child is often to remind her of your unconditional love as you express your opinion. This gives your child space to make her own decisions and makes it more likely that she will ask you for advice as she grows.

Letting go

Letting go is perhaps the hardest part of the parenting process, especially when it comes to sexual decisions. As much as you educate and support your child, in the end, he might make choices that you don't agree with. Whether this involves not waiting to have sex, having more than one partner at a time, or not engaging in safer sex, there comes a time when you no longer have a say in what your child chooses to do with his own body.

While every parent hopes that they have given their teen the tools they need in order to make smart decisions, sometimes people have to make their own mistakes. Your teenager might insist that he is ready to have sex—and it might not be until months later that he regrets his decision and realizes that you were right when you encouraged him to wait. Stepping back and allowing these mistakes to happen isn't easy, but there is nothing else a parent can really do. As generations of parents have discovered, adding rules and regulations will not prevent your child from making certain decisions—they will just ensure that whatever choices he makes are acted out in secret.

If you are having trouble letting go and relinquishing control, it might be a good idea to look inward and identify exactly what you are struggling with. Are you upset purely because your teenager is having sex? Or are you upset that the neighbors might find out and think less of him, or of you as a parent? Are you afraid to let your child grow up, or worried that he will make the same mistakes that you did? Once you have identified the root of your concern, you can move forward and begin to parent your child as effectively as possible in this new stage. In the end, your happiness can't come from your child's decisions, and you have to find a way to come to terms with his new adulthood.

Supporting your child

It can be difficult to support your teen's relationship if she is engaging in sexual activity that you find inappropriate. However, this is a crucial time in the parent-child relationship. If you choose to critique or isolate yourself from the relationship, you risk pushing your child further away. If you don't think that your child is ready to be sexually active, or if you think that she is in a bad relationship, this is a time when you need to give her the most support and unconditional love. A good way to do this is to make it clear that you will always support her, though you cannot always support or agree with her decisions. If your parental intuition is right and she is headed down a bad path with her choice in partner, then you need to be there to help pick up the pieces when it falls apart.

The best way to show your support—without necessarily showing support for the relationship—is to offer her words of encouragement and let her know that she can come talk to you whenever she wants. Make it clear that you want to listen to her even during times when you disagree with her decisions.

For example, you might say: "I know I have said in the past that I think your boyfriend is too old for you. While I do think you should be dating someone your own age, I am still your mother and I want to be here for you no matter what. I am always here to listen about anything you are going through, whether it is a personal matter, something that is going on at school or within your relationship. I hope you feel comfortable talking to me about any issues that come up."

If the relationship does seem to be healthy and happy, make an effort to include your child's partner in your life as a family. Invite him to dinner, get to know his parents, be interested in his life and activities, and always treat the relationship with respect. Just a little bit of parental involvement can go a long way in showing your child support and in keeping your parent-child relationship strong and connected.

HOW TO ANSWER QUESTIONS ABOUT FIRST SEXUAL EXPERIENCES

As your child gets older, questions about sex will have a more personal component. Sharing about your mistakes can have a powerful influence on your child—just be sure to tailor your answers based on your child's maturity and age. Ultimately, you can choose to be as open or as reticent as you like—but remember, be honest. Below are some possible answers, though of course these will depend on your personal experience and comfort level.

Q. What was your first time like?
A. "It was not very good actually. I wish I would have waited," or, "It was very special. I waited until I was with someone who really loved me, and it was very romantic."

Q. Did you regret your first time? Were you embarrassed afterward?
A. "I wasn't embarrassed afterward because I knew my partner respected me and thought I was very special."

Q. Does it hurt to have sex for the first time?
A. "When you are ready to have sex, you will be more relaxed and it will be less likely to hurt. But if you aren't ready, you will likely be very tense, and it can be painful. That's why it is important to wait, and also to be with someone whom you trust and who will take his time and make sure you are comfortable."

Q. Did you wait until you were married?
A. "No, I am sorry to say I didn't wait. I had sex before I was ready because I wanted to fit in. It wasn't a good experience for me and I have always regretted it."

Q. How will I know when I am ready to have sex?
A. "Only you can know that. However, it's important to remember that while you might feel ready in the moment, you might regret the decision the next day. This is why it is important to spend a lot of time thinking about the decision beforehand, and talking about it with your partner."

Identifying unhealthy relationships

For teenagers, as for adults, unhealthy relationships can play out through emotional abuse, physical abuse, or both. It is important to stay involved in your child's relationship to a degree that you can gauge what the day-to-day dynamics of the relationship are. If you notice anything of concern, talk to your child about your worries as soon as you can to prevent possible emotional or physical pain.

Signs of an unhealthy relationship

Unhealthy relationships can be either emotionally or physically damaging—and often these go hand in hand. The most obvious signs of an emotionally unhealthy relationship are sustained and damaging personality changes, such as an obvious loss of confidence or frequent, unexplained anger or sadness.

If you notice these signs, ask your child if she has time to talk. Don't force her if she is unwilling—but do ask if there is a later time when she would be open to talking. By considering her feelings and allowing her some control of the situation, you will help her to feel more comfortable and open. If you do talk, don't pinpoint all the blame on her relationship right away, as this may make her defensive. **Start by saying something such as,** "I have noticed that you have seemed upset lately. I hope you know that if there is anything wrong you can come talk to us about it. Are you and Josh doing okay? How is school? Is there something I can do to make you feel better?"

Physical danger signs can be equally tricky to spot. Abusers are often adept in how they abuse their partners—such as by choosing to hurt them in places that are difficult to see, including the sides, back, and thighs. Furthermore, since most abuse victims are ashamed of their situation, they will go to any lengths to hide these signs.

Physical abuse in teenage relationships is a very real danger which parents should be aware of. According to a SAVE—Safe Alternatives to Violent Environments—study, about one in three American high school students have been or will be involved in an abusive relationship. Talk to your teen if you suspect something is wrong—don't wait. If your child won't confide in you, you may want to introduce her to counseling for extra support and a non-partial listener.

Promoting healing

If your child is getting out of an unhealthy relationship, your support is very important during the recovery stage, especially if the relationship involved abuse. If necessary, alert the police and the teachers at your child's school. Although your teenager might be embarrassed or hesitant to tell anyone about what has happened, assure her that her safety has to come first. Also stress how proud you are of her for having the courage and self-respect to leave a relationship that wasn't working. **For example, you might say:** "I am glad that you broke up with Aaron after he cheated on you. Not many girls would have the strength to do something like that, especially someone as young as you. I am so proud of you. What do you think you are going to do differently in your next relationship?"

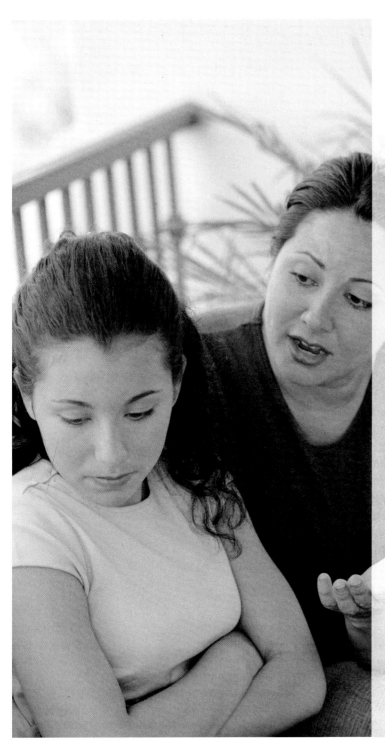

WHAT TO SAY . . .
IF YOU THINK YOUR CHILD IS IN A BAD RELATIONSHIP

If you think that your child is in a bad relationship, your first instinct may be to try to forbid it. However, this tactic has been proven not to work time and time again—not only will your dramatics add to the excitement of the affair, but your child will likely be resourceful enough to find a way to continue the relationship. Instead, try having an open talk about your thoughts and concerns.

CONVERSATION STARTER: "I worry about you spending so much time with Kate. She seems like a nice girl, but she also is a bit of troublemaker."

Allow your child a chance to respond before you go into specifics.

FOLLOW-UP: "I don't want you getting involved with drugs and alcohol, and I also don't like the way she treats you sometimes. I think you should be with a girl who always respects you and treats you well—in the same way you do these things for her."

Once you have expressed your concerns, try to find something to validate about the relationship, then ask specific questions about your child's plans for the future.

FOLLOW-UP: "I know that you have a lot of feelings for Kate, and I am sure she has feelings for you, too, but why do you think you are choosing to be in relationship where you are mistreated? Have you ever wondered why you put up with that? Does it seem difficult sometimes, or does it make you feel sad or hurt?""

Dealing with STDs

STDs are a reality in today's world. Unfortunately, they are often also considered taboo as a discussion topic—which only makes them more scary. It is a good idea to talk openly with your child about STDs from the time you start talking about other serious sexual matters. Staying informed about current research may help you feel more comfortable starting these conversations.

Talking about the realities of STDs

Uncomfortable as it may be, it is essential that your child feels safe talking to you about STDs—more so now than ever, as recent statistics have shown that 1 in 4 teenage girls in the United States has a sexually transmitted disease. Try to start this conversation as early as 9 or 10, when you begin giving more details about sex. Talk about how sexual activity can spread germs, just like sharing a soda or kissing can spread a cold. While it's important not to exaggerate the severity of STDs or try to scare your child, you should emphasize the fact that any type of sexual activity can transmit disease, even if proper protection is worn.

Getting tested

Although you might not want your child to be sexually active, once you know or suspect that he is, it is essential that you promote STD testing. Don't present it as a punishment for his

actions or try to scare him into thinking that he might have an STD. Instead, present it the way you would any other medical or dental appointment—as an important part of caring for your health. Before you do this, it is a good idea to familiarize yourself with the process of testing for STDs, so you can answer any questions your child might have. HIV/AIDS and herpes tests require a blood sample, but other tests are less invasive. For girls, an STD test (including for HPV) can be performed as part of a routine PAP smear.

If your child refuses to go, don't push the issue, but consider asking your family doctor to broach the topic during his next appointment. Your doctor can assure your teen that anything they discuss is confidential, which may make your teen more willing to submit to an STD test or talk about the details of his sexual behavior. **You can encourage your child to get tested** by saying something such as, "I would like to make an appointment at the doctor for you to get an STD test. I will go with you and none of your

"While it's important not to try to scare your child, you should emphasize the fact that any type of sexual activity can transmit disease."

TEACHABLE MOMENT:
TALKING ABOUT STDS

As your child grows, one of the most natural ways to start a conversation about STDs is to share information you learn from studies or media reports. This can encourage discussion without making the topic uncomfortable or too personal. Try saying something such as: "I saw on the news today that 1 in 4 teens has an STD. That really scared me. How does it make you feel? Do you know anyone in your grade with an STD?" Starting these natural conversations can help your child feel more comfortable talking with you about STDs down the road, and might minimize concerns she has about getting in trouble or losing your trust for broaching this topic.

CONVERSATION STARTER 1: "Did you see that article about how common HPV is becoming among teenagers? That is pretty worrying. Are you and your friends aware of facts like that, or is it not talked about very often in your sexual health classes at school?"

CONVERSATION STARTER 2: "It was so scary watching that television program last night where the girl was worried she had an STD after sleeping with her boyfriend. Do you know how and where you can get tested for STDs if you or one of your friends becomes sexually active? It is really important you do this any time you have a new partner."

friends need to know that you are going. It is just for your own peace of mind and to make sure that you are healthy and taking care of yourself. If you want to bring your girlfriend along, I would be happy to drive her as well."

Treating STDs

If your teen finds out that she has an STD, your support can help guide her toward making smarter decisions in the future. It is important not to judge or blame your child for the diagnosis. She is likely already feeling ashamed, and scared, as well as worried about her classmates finding out.

Talk to the doctor so that you can learn about the diagnosis and how it is treated. Make the treatment of the STD as matter-of-fact as you would the treatment of a sore throat or other ailment, but don't forget to also stress the gravity of the situation.

You might say something such as: "I am happy that you were diagnosed with a treatable STD. It's scary to think that there are some STDs that

don't have a cure. I know I probably don't have to tell you to be more careful in the future, but remember that the sexual decisions you make today can follow you throughout your life, so they should be carefully considered."

The good news about STD treatment is that some STDs, such as chlamydia, gonorrhea, and syphilis, can be cured with antibiotics if diagnosed at an early stage. If left untreated, however, they can lead to infertility, pelvic inflammatory disease (PID), and a host of other physical and sexual health issues.

Other STDs, such as HPV and herpes, have no cure. HPV generally clears up on its own within 2 years, but some strains can lead to cervical cancer, or anal cancer in rare cases. Regular exams can help protect your child against this. Herpes outbreaks can be treated with prescription medication. Your child might go months without having an outbreak, but he will still carry the disease. HIV also has no cure, but there are many treatments which can help prolong a person's quality and length of life and help prevent the onset of AIDS.

Learning together

LEARNING ABOUT COMMON STD MYTHS

With so much wrong information being passed around about sexually transmitted diseases, it is hardly surprising that so many young people are becoming infected (two thirds of STDs occur in teenagers and those under 25). Start talking to your child about STDs in her early teens to make sure she has the knowledge she needs to protect herself when she decides to have sex. Use the myths as a springboard for discussion and to help you discover what else your child is curious about.

AFTER THIS LESSON YOUR CHILD WILL BE MORE LIKELY TO...
- Realize the risks involved in any form of sexual contact
- Understand the need to protect herself and her partner
- Have the knowledge she needs to take responsibility for her own health and well-being
- Avoid unsafe sexual behavior
- Know that it is important to see a doctor if she thinks she is at risk
- Understand that unsafe sex now can cause serious problems later in life.

1 ONLY PEOPLE WHO SLEEP AROUND CATCH STDS.

It's true that the more sexual partners you have without using protection, the higher your chances of infection. But you don't have to be promiscuous to get an STD—you can be infected the very first time you have sex—or engage in any form of sexual contact. That's why it is so important to use a condom every time. The only way to ensure that there's no risk of catching an STD is to abstain from sex completely.

2 YOU KNOW WHEN YOU HAVE AN STD BECAUSE YOU HAVE SYMPTOMS.

Sometimes STDs do show symptoms, such as sores or an unusual discharge, but mostly you can't tell whether you or anyone else has an STD. Many infections, including HIV, have no signs and can stay hidden for many years. This is true for both men and women. Chlamydia, which is very common among young people, is another infection that often has no symptoms and it can cause infertility in later life if left untreated. Yet like so many STDs, it can be completely cured if caught at an early stage. If your child thinks she may be at risk, she must see a doctor.

3 YOU CAN'T GET AN STD FROM ORAL SEX

Some STDs, including herpes, can be passed from person to person through oral sex (when you kiss or lick your partner's genitals). For safety, it's best to use a condom or dental dam (a small, thin piece of latex that covers the vulva or anus) during oral sex. There are also STDs, such as herpes and syphilis, which can be spread by skin-to-skin contact. For example, when herpes flares up, a sore appears. When this sore comes into contact with your skin or other moist areas, such as the mouth, throat, and areas with cuts or rashes, it can spread. It can also be spread before the blisters actually form.

4 ONCE YOU'VE HAD AN STD, THERE'S NO CHANCE OF GETTING IT AGAIN

Some STDs, such as herpes and HIV, stay with you for life. Others, like gonorrhea and chlamydia can be treated with antibiotics and completely cured. But you can get infected again if you have sexual contact with anyone who has them. If your child ia diagnosed with an STD, both she and her partner need to be treated so that they don't reinfect each other.

5 IF YOU USE CONDOMS, THERE'S NO CHANCE OF BEING INFECTED.

Using a condom is always important because it helps to prevent the transmission of many STDs, but it does not offer complete protection. Condoms don't cover the entire genital area, so STDs can still be spread by skin-to-skin contact, including HPV and herpes. Because condoms cannot protect against every form of STD, it is important to stress to your child that she should limit the number of sexual partners she has and be tested for STDs on a regular basis.

6 YOU CAN'T GET AN STD FROM MANUAL SEX.

There are risks associated with manual sex just as with any other form of sexual contact. Because it involves skin-to-skin contact, it poses the risk of transmitting bacterial infections such as syphilis, herpes, human papillomavirus (HPV), pubic lice, and scabies. The best way to protect yourself is to wear a latex glove or use a condom during manual sex, and to practice good hand hygiene.

7 TAKING THE ORAL CONTRACEPTIVE PILL PROTECTS AGAINST STDS.

This is probably one of the most common and dangerous misconceptions about STDs. The Pill is a very effective method of birth control when taken correctly, but it offers no protection against STDs whatsoever.

8 GIRLS CAN BE VACCINATED AGAINST STDS

There is a vaccine that is available for girls and young women, but it only helps protect against one STD called HPV, or human papillomavirus. This is a very common virus that affects at least 50 percent of sexually active people at some point in their lives. Often the virus clears on its own. If it persists, it can lead to cervical and other cancers and to genital warts. The vaccine does not protect against all forms of HPV, however, and there are some questions about this relatively new treatment. It is not clear, for example, how it will affect the body's natural immune system, which usually clears most HPV infections on its own. Also, because the vaccine is new, it is possible that other problems or side effects could come to light in the future. Young women can only be vaccinated before they are 26 years old.

HOW TO ANSWER QUESTIONS ABOUT COMMON STD MYTHS

Your child might already know more than you realize about STDs, but much of her information could be incorrect. Make sure that you answer your child's questions accurately and as fully as possible so that she can make the right decisions and protect herself.

Q. Can you catch an STD from a toilet seat?
A. In theory it's possible, but highly unlikely. Bacteria and viruses that cause STDs can't survive outside the human body on a surface like a toilet seat for very long, so the risk of infection is minimal.

Q. Can STDs make you infertile?
A. Yes. About 10 percent of women who are infected with gonorrhea or chlamydia will develop pelvic inflammatory disease (PID), an infection of the uterus, fallopian tubes, or ovaries. It typically occurs during the childbearing years and is the major preventable cause of infertility in the US.

Learning together

Dealing with pregnancy

Working through a teenage pregnancy is challenging and painful for both parents and teens. Communication is especially important during this time. From the beginning, it's important to prepare your child for the process of pregnancy, labor, and possibly motherhood, and to talk as openly as possible about the options your child has and about how you can support her in each of these.

Talking openly about pregnancy

An unwanted pregnancy is one of the most terrifying things a teenager can face. While you don't want to minimize the difficulties or encourage your teenager to have unsafe sex, it is a good idea to reassure her that you are capable of hearing anything she has to tell you—even if it is that she is pregnant. One way to do this is to use a media example to start the conversation in a safe and non-personal climate. **Consider saying something such as:** "Remember that show we watched about the teen who was scared to tell her parents that she was pregnant? If something like that ever happened to you, know that I will support you, even if what you have to tell me is difficult. That is what unconditional love is all about."

Discussing options

If your child finds out that she is pregnant—or finds out that he got his girlfriend pregnant—explaining all of the options is important. Especially if it is your daughter that is pregnant, she has a very big decision before her. Let her know that, in the end, her decision is the most important factor in deciding how to handle her pregnancy. She can listen to your opinion, her boyfriend's opinion, and his family's opinion, but encourage her to do what she decides is right.

If your daughter is considering abortion, talk to her about the different types of abortion available. Depending on where you are in your pregnancy, there are different types of procedures. In the first 9 weeks, a medical abortion is an option, otherwise known as the abortion pill. Some medical abortions are administered via injection. Up to the 12-week mark, a D & C (dilation and curettage) can be performed, where the cervix is dilated and the endometrial lining of the uterus is scraped. After 12 weeks, abortions are performed through D & E (dilation and evacuation) in which vacuum aspiration is accompanied with further dilation of the cervix. After 24 weeks, an abortion is no longer an option, unless the health of the mother is at risk or the baby has severe defects.

According to the Guttmacher Institute, less than 1 percent of women who have an abortion have serious physical complications afterward. However, emotional reactions might be quite overpowering. Women who undergo abortions sometimes experience deep regret, shame, depression or anxiety. Explain to your teen that undergoing an abortion isn't merely a simple medical procedure, such as having one's tonsils out. Instead it can come with a myriad of emotional baggage, baggage that, among other things, can affect your teen's ability to enjoy her sexuality as an adult. Stress that abortions should never be used as a form of contraception.

When talking about adoption, assure your child that she will have the ability to choose the family that adopts her baby. Explain that there are two types of adoption—open and closed. In an open adoption, you are usually able to receive updates about your child, including pictures. Some biological parents are even allowed to visit their child in an open adoption. Closed adoptions don't provide any information or contact with your child.

In both open and closed adoptions, adoption services or adoptive parents generally help to pay for medical expenses involving the pregnancy, and sometimes even offer counseling for the birth mother. However, adoption can an be emotionally tumultuous process. Talk to your teen about how scary and hard it can be to give up a baby that has grown and been nourished in your body for nine months.

If your daughter chooses to keep the baby, talk to her about all this decision will entail. Explain how her life will be changed forever, and how things like school, sports, and friends will need to take second place to the child's well-being. It is important that she is able to envision what her life may be like after giving birth.

If your child is the father, explain that the decision to end or keep the pregnancy is ultimately up to the mother. Talk to him about what fatherhood means and how, if she keeps the baby, he will be responsible for helping to provide support. Be prepared for some anger, sadness, and confusion. This is a difficult time for both young parents and their families, but it is best to avoid assigning blame, which will only further complicate the situation. Make the baby the focus during this time, and support both teenagers as they take this leap into adulthood.

HOW TO ANSWER QUESTIONS ABOUT PREGNANCY

Your teenager will likely have unlimited questions if she finds out that she is pregnant, or if he finds out that his girlfriends is pregnant. Let your child know that you are always available to answer these questions, and try to make your answers as positive as possible, without glossing over the realities of the situation and the steps ahead.

Q. How badly does childbirth hurt?
A. Giving birth is painful, but the doctor will help you be as comfortable as possible. With modern medicine such as epidurals, childbirth can be much less painful than it used to be. And remember that I will be with you every step of the way.

Q. How am I going to finish school and go to college?
A. This will be difficult, but there a lot of schools that have evening and online courses you could attend. It might take you a little longer than other teens your age, but you can achieve this if you work hard.

Q. Should I give my baby up for adoption?
A. I can't decide that for you. In the end this is your baby—and the best thing for both of you is for you to make an informed decision about what is best for your child.

Q. Will my body go back to normal?
A. Pregnancy and childbirth can take a toll on a woman's body, and there is no denying it. However, you are young and healthy, and there is no reason you can't feel comfortable in your own skin after childbirth.

Encouraging safer sex

Even after your child has made the decision to become sexually active, there are still important sexual health lessons to be taught. Talk about the meaning and significance of monogamy, as well as the option to make a second decision for abstinence. It is important that your child realizes that even after he has made the big step to become sexually active, he can protect and cherish his sexuality.

Discussing monogamy

Next to abstinence, monogamy is the safest decision that your teen can make sexually and emotionally. When parenting a sexually active child, try not to lose sight of this. Teens in monogamous relationships can learn important life lessons about responsibility and commitment, even if you don't agree with the sexual decisions they are making. Coming to terms with the realities of your teen's sexual activity involves encouraging him to practice both safer sex and monogamy. In fact, the two are inseparable. This means that although many teenagers want to date and explore sexuality as much as possible, it is important that you suggest that his explorations take a more limited route. To do this, talk to your child about monogamy, since it may not be something that is valued among his friends and peers.

For example, you might say: "You seem to have been dating a lot lately. I want you to enjoy being young and having as much fun as you can, but remember, the fun can end if you aren't safe. I know it's scary to think about, but with all the STDs out there these days, monogamy is the only way to enjoy sex safely. Even condoms can't prevent all STDs. Remember that if you want to be sexually active with someone, even if you decide to be monogamous, you should both get an STD test and get a clean bill of health."

Abstinence after sex

Once someone makes a decision to be sexually active, returning to abstinence can be very difficult, as it might feel pointless or empty. Even if your child regrets her decision to become sexually active, she might feel that returning to a relationship without sex would be meaningless, childish, or trivial. Still, it is a good idea to let her know this is an option. If you feel strongly that it was a mistake for her to jump into sexual activity, encourage your teen to "re-start" her sexual history, so to speak, and return to abstinence. Though she cannot erase the decision to lose her virginity, she can make a healthy decision to wait until she is older to continue having sex.

To start this conversation, talk with your child about how sexual health and sexual worth do not stem from having sex one time, or even from having sex numerous times. Let her know that respecting your body and your sexuality means abstaining from sex until you are ready, whether or not you have already had sex.

Try saying something such as: "I know we have talked about how you wished you would have waited to have sex. However, you can still abstain from sex, and that can be a meaningful decision. Just because you made a mistake one time, that is no justification to keep making the same mistake."

Reasserting value

An important part of this conversation is helping your child understand that she is not damaged or less valuable because she has had sex. It is still common for sexual history to be linked to a person's worth, especially for women. When a girl is looked down on or called names by her peers because she has had sex, she might think that she is condemned to have that reputation, and thus decide to continue having sex. Even though she secretly hates being mistreated by her classmates, she might prefer to act aloof or casual about sex. She may even pretend to enjoy her reputation, just so that no one can see how deeply her feelings are hurt.

Help heal these painful feelings by talking to your teen about how no one has the right to judge her sexual decisions—nor does she have the right to judge anyone else's. Having this conversation can help empower your teen to abstain from sex, and can also help her realize that her sexual decisions are personal, not public. Once she is able to disentangle her self-worth from what other children at school say about her, or from any mistakes she might have made in the past, she will be more likely to make choices for her own personal happiness and security. This means that she will be less likely to engage in promiscuous behavior in an attempt to gain attention or popularity, and that she will not think of her body as a commodity to be bartered or used casually.

You might start by saying: "It seems like you have been having kind of a hard time at school since you and John made the decision to have sex. Do any of the kids at school say things that make you regret your decision? No matter what they say, know that having sex does not change who you are as a person."

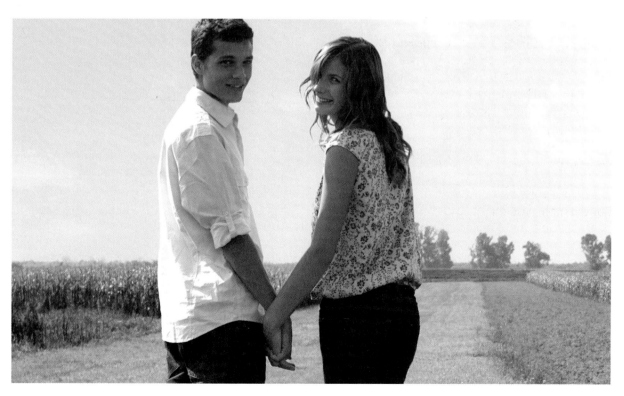

Glossary

Use this list of terms to help define words that are new to you or that you may have difficulty explaining to your child. Referring back to these concise definitions can help you grasp terms that might otherwise seem overwhelming or intimidating.

abortion
The purposeful termination of a pregnancy using surgical techniques or drugs.

acquaintance rape
Rape by someone who is already known to the victim.

AIDS
Acquired Immune Deficiency Syndrome. A disease that causes the breakdown of the immune system, making people vulnerable to opportunistic infections and some types of cancer. AIDS is caused by the Human Immunodeficiency Virus (HIV).

anorexia nervosa
An eating disorder in which people severely restrict their food intake or starve themselves, resulting in an extremely low body weight.

bulimia nervosa
An eating disorder characterized by uncontrollable binge eating followed by compensatory behavior, such as fasting or self-induced vomiting.

cap
A barrier method of contraception for women. A cap is inserted into the vagina to cover the cervix prior to sexual intercourse. Also known as a diaphragm.

chlamydia
A common bacterial STD. Girls and women with chlamydia often have no symptoms. Boys and men usually have a discharge and pain when urinating.

circumcision
The surgical removal of the foreskin from the penis, which may be performed for cultural or medical reasons.

clitoris
Part of the female genitals, located just below the pubic bone; the main organ of female sexual arousal.

closed adoption
A type of adoption in which there is minimal or no contact between biological and adoptive parents.

concrete operational stage
A developmental stage of childhood (age 6–12) in which a child begins to think logically, solve problems, and understand the views and feelings of others. In this stage your child no longer has an ego-centric viewpoint.

condom
A barrier method of contraception, usually made of latex. The male condom is a sheath that is unrolled onto the erect penis prior to intercourse. The female condom is inserted into the vagina prior to intercourse.

contraceptive pill
A hormonal method of contraception for women, which is taken orally, usually on a daily basis. Also commonly known as "The Pill."

date rape
Rape by someone who is already known to the victim, usually occurring while on a date.

dental dam
A latex or polyurethane barrier designed to prevent the transmission of STDs during oral sex (placed over the genitals/anus of the person receiving oral sex).

dilation and evacuation
A technique used in surgical abortions. The cervix is dilated and the contents of the uterus are removed.

ejaculation
The expulsion of semen from the penis at the peak of sexual arousal. Ejaculation happens when the penis is stimulated during masturbation or intercourse, but can also happen during sleep (called a "nocturnal emission"), or for no apparent reason. Boys begin to have ejaculations as they enter adolescence.

endorphins
Chemicals produced by the pituitary gland in the brain. Endorphins are released at the moment of orgasm, and are responsible for pleasurable feelings.

epidural
A type of anesthetic injected into the epidural space of the spine, used to relieve labor pains during childbirth.

erection
The stiffening and enlargement of the penis and the clitoris during sexual arousal. An erection results from a rush of blood to the genital tissues.

estrogen
The hormone that controls female sexual development and the functioning of the reproductive system.

follicle-stimulating hormone (FSH)
A hormone produced by the pituitary gland in the brain. It stimulates the production of eggs in girls and women.

formal operational stage
A developmental stage in childhood (age 12-15) in which a child becomes capable of abstract thought and has a heightened sense of self-awareness.

gender script
A behavioral script based on what society expects from boys and girls. An example of a behavioral script for boys would be "Boys don't cry."

genital warts
A viral sexually transmitted disease that results in the development of warts around the genital area.

genitals
The external reproductive organs in men and women.

gonadotropin-releasing hormone (GnRH)
A hormone that stimulates the pituitary gland to release follicle-stimulating hormone and luteinizing hormone.

gonorrhea
A bacterial sexually transmitted disease that can be treated with antiobiotics. Gonorrhea may be symptomless or it may cause a vaginal or penile discharge.

herpes
A viral sexually transmitted disease that results in painful blisters and sores on the genitals. The herpes virus can also cause cold sores on the lips and mouth.

HIV
Human Immunodeficiency Virus, the virus that causes Acquired Immune Deficiency Syndrome (AIDS). HIV can be transmitted through unprotected sexual intercourse, blood transfusions, or the sharing of non-sterile needles.

homosexuality
Sexual attraction between people of the same sex.

human papilloma virus (HPV)
A virus that causes genital warts, one of the most common sexually transmitted diseases. Some types of HPV are linked with an increased risk of cervical cancer.

implant
A hormonal method of contraception for women. Implants are inserted under the skin of the arm and they release hormones into the body to prevent pregnancy.

intra-uterine device (IUD)
A method of contraception for women in which a T-shaped device is inserted into the uterus. Some IUDs release hormones into the body just as the Pill does; others are non-hormonal.

Kaposi's sarcoma
A type of cancer found in AIDS patients, which causes patches of abnormal tissue to grow under the skin.

labia
The lips that surround the vulva. The hair-covered external lips are the labia majora; the inner hairless lips are the labia minora.

luteinizing hormone (LH)
A hormone produced by the pituitary gland. A surge of LH occurs before ovulation.

masturbation
Sexual self-stimulation of the genitals, usually by hand.

medical abortion
Termination of pregnancy using drugs; sometimes known as "the abortion pill."

menstrual cycle
The sequence of hormonal changes that women experience roughly every 28 days, beginning during puberty and lasting until menopause. During each menstrual cycle an egg is released from the ovary. If the egg isn't fertilized it leaves the body during menstruation, as the lining of the uterus is shed.

menstruation
The shedding of the uterine lining; also known as a monthly period. Blood flow and other side effects usually last between three to seven days.

menopause
The point at which a woman ceases producing eggs and is no longer able to conceive, usually in late middle age. Menstruation ends as a result of falling hormone levels.

negative feedback
A behavioral management technique in which a person is given an explanation of what they have done wrong and how they can fix it. It's used as a more constructive alternative to criticism, insults, and aggression.

nocturnal emission
Ejaculation that takes place while a boy or man is asleep; also known as a "wet dream." This is common during adolescence.

open adoption
A type of adoption in which the biological parent can receive information about the child or sometimes even retain contact with the child as he grows up.

orgasm
The climax or peak of sexual pleasure.

ovaries
Female reproductive organs in which egg follicles are stored. An egg is released from an ovary in each menstrual cycle.

ovulation
The moment at which an egg or ovum is released from an ovary (part of the menstrual cycle).

oxytocin
A hormone that's released after orgasm and bonds two people together by producing feel-good emotions. Also known as the "cuddle chemical."

Pap test
A screening test for cervical cancer. Cells are collected from the outer opening of the cervix and examined for pre-cancerous changes.

parallel play
A type of play in which young children enjoy playing alongside each other but don't interact with each other directly. This usually happens around two years of age.

patch
A hormonal method of contraception for women. A patch is stuck to the skin and it releases hormones into the body that help prevent pregnancy.

pelvic inflammatory disease (PID)
An infection of the female reproductive system, often as a result of sexually transmitted diseases such as chlamydia. Infertility can be a complication of PID.

penis
The primary male sex organ, through which urine and semen pass.

pituitary gland
A gland in the brain that produces hormones, including follicle-stimulating hormone and luteinizing hormone. The pituitary gland is know for triggering the start of puberty.

placenta
An organ that develops inside the uterus during pregnancy. It supplies the growing baby with food and oxygen and transports waste products away to be disposed of by the mother's body.

post-ovulatory phase
The phase of the menstrual cycle that takes place after an egg has been released from the ovary.

preoperational stage
A developmental stage in which a child (age 2–6) is egocentric in nature and thinks on a fantasy level.

pre-ejaculate
The sperm-containing fluid that appears at the head of the penis during sexual arousal, just before orgasm.

pre-ovulatory phase
The phase of a girl's or woman's menstrual cycle that takes place in the build-up to egg release (ovulation).

progesterone
A female hormone that's released by the ovary after an egg is released in each menstrual cycle. Progesterone is also produced by the placenta during pregnancy.

puberty
The period of sexual maturation that usually takes place in the early teens, though it can begin anywhere between 9–15 years of age. Puberty is initiated by hormones. During puberty, a child's body develops into an adult body and becomes capable of reproduction.

pubic lice
Small parasites that attach themselves to the pubic hair and reproduce by laying eggs. Also known as "crabs." They can be transmitted through sexual contact or contact with infested bedding or clothing.

safer sex
Sexual behavior that reduces the risk of pregnancy and of transmitting STDs; for example, by wearing a male or female condom. Also known as protected sex.

scrotum
The bag or pouch that hangs below the penis and contains the testes.

semen
The sperm-containing fluid that is released from the penis at the moment of ejaculation.

sensorimotor stage
A developmental stage in childhood (from birth to the age of 2) in which a child is primarily focused on sensation and movement.

sexting
Sending or receiving sexually explicit messages, pictures, or videos, generally by cell phone.

sperm
The male sex cells produced by the testes. Sperm production begins at the start of puberty and lasts the rest of an adult male's life. A single sperm cell fertilizes an egg during fertilization.

spermicide
A method of contraception that comes in the form of creams, jellies, foams, films, and pessaries. Spermicide can be used on its own or with the sponge, diaphragm, or cap.

sponge
A barrier method of contraception. The sponge is inserted into the vagina prior to sexual intercourse.

STD
Sexually transmitted disease. An STD may be viral, such as herpes; bacterial, such as gonorrhea; or parasitic, such as pubic lice.

suction curettage
A technique used in surgical abortions, where suction is used to empty the contents of the uterus. Also known as vacuum aspiration.

surgical abortion
Termination of pregnancy using surgical techniques such as dilation and evacuation.

syphilis
A bacterial sexually transmitted disease that has several stages, the first of which is an appearance of a sore known as a "chancre."

testes
The sperm-producing organs that are held in the scrotum.

testosterone
The main male sex hormone. It stimulates sexual development at puberty and controls the male reproductive system and sex drive.

toxic shock syndrome
A rare condition that may be caused by using tampons. Symptoms include high fever, rash, and a sudden drop in blood pressure.

trichomoniasis
A common vaginal infection that causes discharge and inflammation. Trichomoniasis can be easily treated with antibiotics, though you can catch it again once cured.

urinary tract infection (UTI)
A bacterial infection in any part of the urinary system. The most common UTI in women is cystitis, an inflammation of the bladder.

uterus
A female reproductive organ situated above the vagina. It expands massively to accommodate the growing fetus during pregnancy.

urethra
A tube that transfers urine from the urinary bladder to outside the body. In men it passes through the penis. In women it is situated above the vaginal opening.

vagina
The muscular passage that's part of the female reproductive system. The vagina is penetrated by the penis during intercourse, it acts as a birth canal, and it channels menstrual blood out of the body.

vulva
The external female genitals; includes the clitoris, labia, and urethral and vaginal entrances.

Bibliography

Each of the works cited below was referenced in this book. Together, these comprise some of the most informative and groundbreaking research conducted about sexual education and health in recent years. Refer to these tools as needed for more in-depth information or statistics about a given topic.

Chapter 1: Talking about the body

Anderson, Sarah E. and Whitaker, Robert C. "The Prevalence of Obesity Among US Preschool Children in Different Racial and Ethnic Groups." **Archives of Pediatrics and Adolescent Medicine,** Ohio State University (April 2009).

Kilbourne, Jean. **Slim Hopes.** VHS. Media Education Foundation, 1995.

National Sleep Foundation. 2009. "How Much Sleep Do We Really Need?" http://www.sleepfoundation.org/how-much-sleep-do-we-really-need.

Ouyang, F. et al. "Serum DDT, Age at Menarche, and Abnormal Menstrual Cycle Length." **Occupational and Environmental Medicine** 62, no. 12 (2005): 878-884.

Women's Sports Foundation. 2008. "Go Out and Play: Youth Sports in America." http://www.womenssportsfoundation.org/Content/Research-Reports/Go-Out-and-Play.aspx.

Chapter 2: Talking about the mind

Cantor, J.M. et al. "How Many Gay Men Owe Their Sexual Orientation to Fraternal Birth Order." **Archives of Sexual Behavior** 31, no. 1 (2002): pp. 63-71.

Diamond, Lisa M. et al. "Development of sexual orientation among adolescent and young adult women." **Developmental Psychology** (January 2000).

Kinsey, Alfred et al. **Sexual Behavior of the Human Male.** Philadelphia: W. B. Saunders Company (1948).

Kinsey, Alfred et al. **Sexual Behavior of the Human Female.** Philadelphia: W. B. Saunders Company (1953).

Piaget, Jean and Inhelder, B. **The Psychology of the Child.** New York: Basic Books (1962).

University of Illinois at Chicago. "In Fruit Flies, Homosexuality is Biological But Not Hard-Wired, Study Shows." **ScienceDaily** December 10, 2007. http://www.sciencedaily.com/releases/2007/12/071210094541.htm/.

Chapter 3: Talking about the media

Groesz, Lisa M. et al. "The Effect of Experimental Presentation of Thin Media Images on Body Satisfaction: A Meta-Analytic Review." **International Journal of Eating Disorders** 31 (2002).

Hofschire, L.J., and Greenberg, B.S. "Media's Impact on Adolescents' Body Dissatisfaction." In J.D. Brown, J.R. Steele, and K. Walsh-Childers (Eds) **Sexual Teens, Sexual Media.** NJ: Lawrence Erlbaum Associates, Inc.

Klein, Hugh and Shiffman, Kenneth. "Thin is 'In' and Stout is 'Out': What Animated Cartoons Tell Viewers About Body Weight." Paper presented at the annual meeting of the American Sociological Association, Hilton San Francisco & Renaissance Parc 55 Hotel, San Francisco, CA, Aug 14, 2004.

Liz Claiborne Inc. study on teen dating abuse conducted by Teenage Research Unlimited (February 2005).

Mccabe, Marita P. and Vincent, Maureen A. "Development of Body Modification and Excessive

Exercise Scales for Adolescents." **Assessment** 9, no. 2 (June 2002).

Primack, Brian et al. "Exposure to Sexual Lyrics and Sexual Experience Among Urban Adolescents." **American Journal of Preventative Medicine** 36, no. 4 (April 2009).

Chapter 4: Talking about friends and influences

Blum RW and Rinehart PM. 2000. "Protecting Teens: Beyond Race, Income and Family Structure." Minneapolis: Division of General Pediatrics & Adolescent Health, University of Minnesota Adolescent Health Program (2000).

Clark, Sheila. "Parents, peers, and pressures: Identifying the influences on responsible sexual decision-making." **Adolescent Health, Practice Update from the National Association of Social Workers** 2, no. 2 (September 2001), http://www.socialworkers. org/practice/adolescent_health/ah0202.asp/.

Chapter 6: Talking about sexual relationships

Centers for Disease Control and Prevention. 2008. "Genital HPV Infection," CDC fact sheet, http://www. cdc.gov/STD/HPV/STDFact-HPV.htm/.

Centers for Disease Control and Prevention. 2008. "HIV/AIDS Among Youth." http://www.cdc.gov/hiv/ resources/factsheets/youth.htm/.

Centers for Disease Control and Prevention. 2006. "HIV Prevalence Estimates, United States." http://www. cdc.gov/mmwr/preview/mmwrhtml/mm5739a2.htm/.

Centers for Disease Control and Prevention, 2007. "Sexually Transmitted Disease Surveillance, Chlamydia." http://www.cdc.gov/std/stats07/ chlamydia.htm/.

Centers for Disease Control and Prevention. 2007. "Sexually Transmitted Disease Surveillance, Gonorrhea." http://www.cdc.gov/std/stats07/ gonorrhea.htm/.

Centers for Disease Control and Prevention. 2007. "Sexually Transmitted Disease Surveillance, Syphilis." http://www.cdc.gov/std/stats07/syphilis.htm.

Centers for Disease Control and Prevention. 2007. "Trichomoniasis," CDC fact sheet, http://www.cdc.gov/ STD/Trichomonas/STDFact-Trichomoniasis.htm/.

Kohler, Pamela. "Abstinence-Only and Comprehensive Sex Education and the Initiation of Sexual Activity and Teen Pregnancy." **Journal of Adolescent Health** (April 2008).

Langer, Gary, "ABC News Poll: Sex Lives of American Teens," **ABCNews.go.com,** May 19, 2006, http:// abcnews.go.com/Primetime/PollVault/ story?id=1981945&page=1/.

"Florida teens believe drinking bleach will prevent HIV," **Local6.com,** April 2, 2008, http://www. clickorlando.com/news/15773787/detail.html.

Planned Parenthood. 2009. Birth Control, http://www. plannedparenthood.org/health topics/birth-control-4211.htm.

Prinstein, Mitchell J. "Adolescent Oral Sex, Peer Popularity, and Perceptions of Best Friends' Sexual Behavior." **Journal of Pediatric Psychology** 28, no. 4 (June 2003).

Sessions Stepp, Laura, "Study: Half of All Teens Have Had Oral Sex," **Washington Post,** September 16, 2005.

UNAIDS. 2008. "Report on the global AIDS epidemic." http://www.unaids.org/en/KnowledgeCentre/HIVData/ GlobalReport/2008/2008_Globalreport.asp/.

Wight, Daniel et al: "The Quality of Young People's Heterosexual Relationships: A Longitudinal Analysis of Characteristics Shaping Subjective Experience." **Perspectives on Sexual and Reproductive Health** (December 2008).

Further resources

The following books and websites provide further information for you and your child about all aspects of sexual education. You may like to read through books before passing them to your children to make sure the advice they contain is in keeping with your own values and beliefs. You might also wish to introduce these sex education resources to your child's school.

Organizations and websites

Centers for Disease Control and Prevention
www.cdc.gov

ChildHelp (National Child Abuse Hotline)
www.childhelp.org

Get in Touch
www.getintouchfoundation.org

Guttmacher Institute
www.guttmacher.org

Life in the Fast Lane
www.teenageparent.org

Love is Respect (National Teen Dating Abuse Hotline)
www.loveisrespect.org

Nitestar
www.nitestar.org

PFLAG (Parents, Families, and Friends of Lesbians and Gays
www.pflag.org

Planned Parenthood
www.plannedparenthood.org

SIECUS (Sex Information Education Council of the United States)
www.siecus.org

Books for children

Changing bodies, changing lives: a book for teens on sex and relationships
by Ruth Bell
(Three Rivers Press 1998)

What's going on down there? Answers to questions boys find hard to ask
by Karen Gravelle et al
(Walker Books 1998)

It's perfectly normal: changing bodies, growing up, sex, and sexual health
by Robie H. Harris
(Candlewick 2004)

It's so amazing! A book about eggs, sperm, birth, babies, and families
by Robie H. Harris
(Candlewick 2004)

What's happening to me?
by Peter Mayle
(Lyle Stuart 2000)

Where did I come from?
by Peter Mayle
(Lyle Stuart 2000)

Our bodies, ourselves: a new edition
for a new era
by Judy Norsigian
(Touchstone 2005)

The care & keeping of you: the body
book for girls
by Valorie Schaefer
(American Girl Publishing 1998)

Bellybuttons are navels
by Mark Schoen
(BookSurge 2008)

Books for parents

Teaching your children healthy sexuality: a
biblical approach to preparing them for life
by Jim Burns
(Bethany House 2008)

From diapers to dating: A parent's guide to
raising sexually healthy children
by Debra W. Haffner
(Newmarket 2008)

What every 21st-century parent needs to know:
facing today's challenges with wisdom and heart
by Debra W. Haffner
(Newmarket 2008)

Everything you never wanted your kids to know
about sex, but were afraid they'd ask: the
secrets to surviving your child's sexual
development from birth to the teens
by Justin Richardson and Mark A. Schuster
(Three Rivers Press 2004)

Index

London, New York, Melbourne, Munich, and Delhi

Editors Ross Hilton, Daniel Mills, Jimmy Topham
Senior Art Editor Sara Robin
US Editor Shannon Beatty
Executive Managing Editor Adèle Hayward
Managing Art Editor Kat Mead
Senior Production Editor Jennifer Murray
Creative Technical Support Sonia Charbonnier
Senior Production Controller Man Fai Lau
Art Director Peter Luff
Publisher Stephanie Jackson

Produced for Dorling Kindersley by
Project Editor Nichole Morford
Designers Emma and Tom Forge

First American Edition, 2009

Published in the United States by
DK Publishing
375 Hudson Street
New York, NY 10014
09 10 11 10 9 8 7 6 5 4 3 2 1
175554-September 2009

Published in Great Britain by
Dorling Kindersley Limited.

A catalog record of this book is available from the
Library of Congress:
ISBN: 978-0-7566-5738-3

DK books are available at special discounts when
purchased in bulk for sales promotions, premiums,
fund-raising, or educational use. For details,
contact: DK Publishing Special Markets, 375
Hudson Street, New York, NY 10014, or
SpecialSales@dk.com.

Printed and bound in USA by RR Donnelley

Discover more at www.dk.com

This book is dedicated to my three boys, Ethan, Sammy, and Jackson, who have been my greatest students, but more so my most brilliant teachers. I love you oodles and oodles of noodles.

Author Acknowledgments There are so many people who have made this book possible. It's a subject that has been near and dear to my heart for so long. I want to thank Dorling Kindersley Publishing, especially Stephanie Jackson and Nichole Morford, as well as my agent, Binky Urban, for being willing to address this crucial but often touchy subject, and for allowing me to voice my often controversial perspectives! Nick Kahn at ICM Talent, thank you for working so tirelessly on my behalf and for being so supportive and fun along the way. Thank you to everyone at Harpo, especially Ms. Winfrey for giving me the amazing opportunities to put my ideas on sex education out to the world, Erik Logan for helping to make it all happen with amazing humor and kindness, and Corny Koehl, Alicia Haywood, Matthew Commings, Scott Clifton, and the rest of the team at Oprah Radio who are masters at what they do and who so smoothly and creatively make it possible for me to host the *Dr. Laura Berman Show* live every day! Thank you also to Empower Public Relations for your constant attention to getting my voice heard. Also a big thank you to my managers at ROAR, especially Greg Suess. And thank you, thank you to Bridget Sharkey, you are a phenomenal machine of endless energy and your willingness to work under the gun to get this book finished is so appreciated! You are so quiet on the outside and such a powerhouse on the inside! I also want to give a special thank you and shout to Dr. Cydelle Berlin and Nitestar (formally Star Theater) who gave me my first introduction to sex education in graduate school and helped set the foundation and inspiration for my passion and dedication to educating children about their bodies and their sexuality. You do such amazing work and I hope your efforts spread around the world.

 Thank you also to my parents Linda and Irwin Berman for modeling for me what it is to be comfortable and open about sexuality. You set the bar high for how to raise a sexually healthy child and I learned from the masters. To my husband Sam, thank you for being my life, love, and creative partner, and for joining with me in our quest to raise three sexually healthy, respectful, and empowered sons. I know you are the one that always seems to get the tough questions and you always handle them with aplomb and in a way that makes me proud and thankful to call you my co-parent.

DK Acknowledgments Thanks to Steve Crozier for retouching work, Rebecca Warren for proofreading, Marie Lorimer for indexing, Harriet Mills and Jo Walton for picture research, and Tom Howells, Kesta Desmond, and Mandy Lebentz for their invaluable help with editorial work.

Picture Credits Illustrations by Mark Watkinson. The publisher would like to thank the following for their kind permission to reproduce their photographs:
(Key: a-above; b-below/bottom; c-center; f-far; l-left; r-right; t-top)

Alamy Images: Science Photo Library/Ian Hooton 163; **Corbis:** 81A Productions 57; Ephraim Ben-Shimon 171; Frederic Cirou/PhotoAlto 167; Goodshoot 43; Image Source 81; KMSS 4ftl; Kate Mitchell 165; George Shelley 2; Stockbyte 4tr, 54-55; Thinkstock 65; **Getty Images:** Jenny Acheson 116-117; Janie Airey 179; Tony Anderson 61; Barry Austin Photography 113; Hans Bjurling 5ftr, 160-161; Felix Clinton 67; John Cumming 15; Jim Cummins 53; Digital Vision 8-9, 73; Flying Colours Ltd 21, 78-79; Gallo Images/ Richard Keppel-Smith 151; George Shelley Productions 125; Jamie Grill 133; Image Source 41, 143; Jose Luis Pelaez Inc 91; Jupiterimages 5ftl, 11, 105, 115; Sean Justice 93, 103; Johannes Kroemer 159; Titus Lacoste 1, 5tl; Ryan McVay/Photodisc 99; Sean Murphy 141; PhotoAlto/Laurence Mouton 13; Photolibrary 35; Justin Pumfrey 5tr, 136-137; Christopher Robbins 100-101; Andersen Ross 31; Richard Schultz 121; Stockbyte 4ftr, 89; SW Productions 155; Tetra Images 4tl, 17; Katja Zimmermann 109; **Photolibrary:** Comstock Images 131, 135; Creatas 139; Ryan McVay 77; Monkey Business Images Ltd 119.

All other images © Dorling Kindersley
For further information see: www.dkimages.com